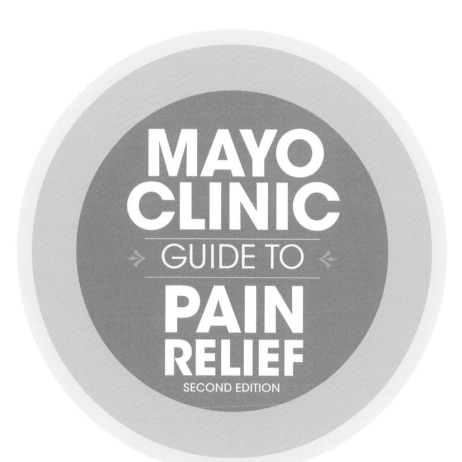

MAYO
CLINIC
→ GUIDE TO ←
PAIN
RELIEF
SECOND EDITION

Barbara K. Bruce, Ph.D.
Tracy E. Harrison, M.D.

Medical Editors

Mayo Clinic
Rochester, Minnesota

Mayo Clinic Guide to Pain Relief provides reliable, practical information on managing chronic pain. Much of the information comes directly from the experience of pain specialists and other health care professionals at Mayo Clinic. This book supplements the advice of your physician, whom you should consult for individual medical problems.

For bulk sales to employers, member groups and health-related companies, contact Mayo Clinic Health Solutions, 200 First St. SW, Rochester, MN, 55905, or send an e-mail to SpecialSalesMayoBooks@Mayo.edu.

Published by Mayo Clinic

© 2013 Mayo Foundation for Medical Education and Research (MFMER)

Library of Congress Control Number: 2013941413

Second Edition

1 2 3 4 5 6 7 8 9 10

Image credits

Editorial staff

Preface

To maintain good health and manage illness, it's important to have helpful and reliable information. This is particularly true for the common and often-complicated problem of chronic pain.

Advances in the field of pain medicine continue to occur at a rapid pace. This new edition of *Mayo Clinic Guide to Pain Relief* includes the most recent information on how the nervous system responds to painful illness and injury and common pain conditions such as low back pain, migraines and fibromyalgia.

The pain management strategies presented in this book are based on the expertise of Mayo Clinic physicians, psychologists, nurses, and physical and occupational therapists. We are indebted to the staff of Mayo Clinic's Pain Rehabilitation Center, Pain Clinic and Fibromyalgia Treatment Program for their guidance and assistance.

We believe you'll find this book to be a helpful and practical resource for effectively managing your pain and finding the relief you seek.

Barbara K. Bruce, Ph.D.
Tracy E. Harrison, M.D.
Medical Editors

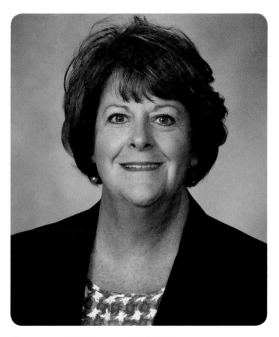

Barbara K. Bruce, Ph.D.

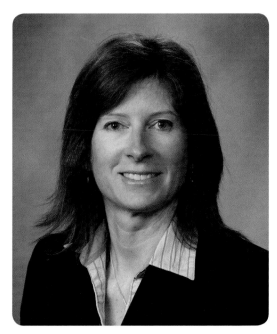

Tracy E. Harrison, M.D.

Table of contents

Part 3: Managing chronic pain............................ 159

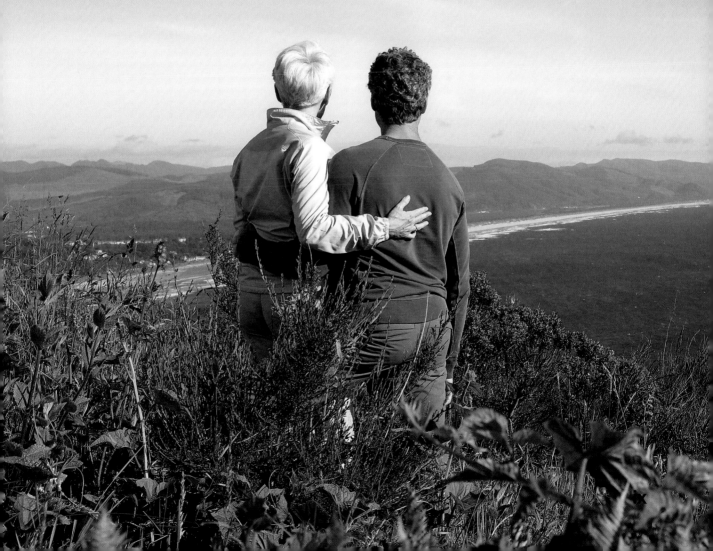

Part 1

Understanding chronic pain

Chapter 1

About this book

When you're in pain, there's nothing you want more than relief from the constant throbbing, stinging or aching. With many types of injuries and illnesses, given time, the pain will eventually disappear. But not all pain can be eliminated. For some people, the pain never goes away. Does this mean you can never experience pain relief? No, it doesn't. But it does mean you may have to change your definition of relief.

With some types of chronic, or persistent, pain, medications and interventions are available that can produce a major reduction in pain, and possibly even get rid of the pain altogether. In other instances, however, nothing seems to work. No matter what the treatment — pills, a shot, surgery — the pain endures. But even in this

situation, you can still experience pain relief. Given the right tools and techniques, you can reduce the aching and throbbing to a more tolerable level — one that you can live with.

Mayo Clinic Guide to Pain Relief is a comprehensive, how-to pain control manual. Whether you've lived with chronic pain for years or have recently been diagnosed, this book can supply you with the information and tools to minimize and manage your pain. Our hope is that this book will make you a better consumer of medical care for your pain, regardless of the type of pain you're experiencing or how long you've been searching for pain relief.

While the focus of this book is on the treatment of chronic pain, we also provide up-to-date information on treatments used to control short-term (acute) pain that follows surgery or an accident, such as a broken bone.

Why is managing pain important? Pain can interfere with your enjoyment of life. It can make it difficult to sleep, work, socialize with friends and family, and accomplish everyday tasks. When your ability to function is limited, you may become less productive. Ongoing pain can cause you to lose your appetite and feel weak and depressed. You may also find yourself avoiding hobbies and other enjoyable activities in order to prevent further injury or pain. But while your pain may be part of you, it doesn't have to destroy you.

By learning how to manage your pain, you can reclaim your life and become some or all of the person that you used to be. This book is about helping you find the relief you seek.

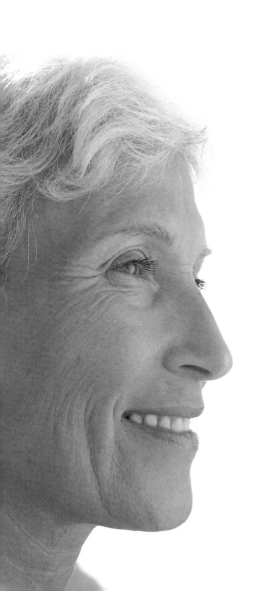

How to use this book

Mayo Clinic Guide to Pain Relief emphasizes a take-charge approach to successfully managing chronic pain by providing detailed information and instructions on a variety of strategies for controlling pain. These include daily exercise, activity modification, stress-reduction techniques, behavior changes and goal setting. The book also discusses when medications may be useful and why many times medications aren't the answer to long-term pain control.

Your level of pain and how much it's affecting your ability to function will

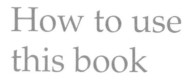

determine how best to use this book. If you've just begun to experience persistent pain, you may find the discussion of how pain develops and various treatments for chronic pain most helpful. If you've been battling chronic pain for years and have concluded that medications don't help or they cause unwanted side effects, the last section of the book on pain management strategies can teach you how to better manage your pain without medication.

However, regardless of your pain type or its severity, the best way to use this book and to gain the most from it is to read it from beginning to end — and return to it as needed.

The three parts

Mayo Clinic Guide to Pain Relief is divided into three sections, or parts. The first section provides valuable background to help you better understand why you're in pain. The second section focuses on medical treatments and therapies that can help control pain. The third section is the "what you can do" portion of the book. This section addresses specific steps you can take to help relieve your pain.

Part 1: Understanding chronic pain

To control your pain, you need to understand how pain develops, what influences pain and why some pain persists. Part 1 discusses the anatomy of pain — the parts of your body involved in the development of pain — and why some people respond to pain differently than do others. There's also information on conditions and illnesses commonly associated with chronic pain, as well as a discussion of the long-term physical, emotional and financial effects of ongoing pain.

Part 2: Treating chronic pain

There are many options for treating pain. The most common is medication. Part 2 begins with a discussion of various drugs used to relieve pain. You can learn why some medications are generally more effective for certain types of pain than are others. You'll also read about the potential side effects of some pain medications, especially if the drugs are taken in large doses or over the long term.

In addition, Part 2 reviews other types of treatments used to relieve pain, such as injections given at pain sites, nerve stimulators and medication pumps, as well as alternative and complementary therapies. If you're considering seeing a pain specialist or your primary care doctor has recommended that you do so, there's a discussion of the different types of pain clinics, centers and programs available and what to look for to find the right one for you.

Part 3: Managing chronic pain

With chronic pain, there often isn't an effective medication used alone that can completely eliminate your pain. The next step then becomes learning how to live with the pain.

Part 3 focuses on steps you can take to manage your pain so that it doesn't interfere with your ability to work, spend time with family and friends, or enjoy life. And what people have found is that when their pain is no longer the focus of their attention, its severity tends to decrease.

Some of the strategies for managing chronic pain discussed in Part 3 include goal setting, daily exercise, activity modification, emotional and behavioral changes, positive thinking, stress management, sleep improvement, healthy eating, weight control and improved family relationships.

Part 3 is where you'll find information on steps that you can take on your own to get yourself on course to life with less pain.

Chapter 2

What is pain?

Pain is a universal experience. We all feel it, whether it's the sharp, stabbing pain of a twisted ankle or the deep, throbbing pain of a headache that won't quit. Pain knows no age limit — it affects us from infancy through old age. Approximately 1 in 3 Americans reports experiencing at least one episode of persistent pain.

What exactly is pain? Pain is defined as "a localized sensation of discomfort or distress, resulting from the stimulation of specialized nerve endings."

Sensitivity to pain is complex, and it varies from person to person. An experience that may cause one person immediate, excruciating pain may result in only minor discomfort for another. This varied sensitivity can sometimes make pain hard to compare or to evaluate. The degree to which you feel pain and how you react to it are the results of your biological, psychological and cultural makeup. In addition, past encounters with a painful injury or illness can influence your sensitivity to pain.

There are times when pain can be useful — almost protective — such as when it warns you that the hot skillet you've just picked up will burn your hand if you don't put it down quickly. But other pain — the day-after-day chronic ache of arthritis or the constant throbbing of a headache — seems to serve no useful purpose. And its relentlessness can be overwhelming.

When pain persists beyond the time expected for an injury to heal or an illness to end, it can become a chronic condition. No longer is the pain viewed as the symptom of another disease, rather it's seen as an illness unto itself. This type of pain is known as chronic pain, or chronic noncancer pain in order to distinguish it from cancer (malignant) pain. Other names include chronic pain syndrome or chronic benign pain, although nothing about it may seem benign.

Chronic pain can be difficult to treat. Often, medication alone isn't sufficient to help people who struggle with chronic pain. In most instances, a comprehensive approach is used, which may include medication, physical therapy, psychological and behavioral therapy, and interventional treatments such as injections and nerve blocks.

Making sense of your nervous system

Your nervous system is composed of nerve cells and fibers that transmit and receive messages in the form of electrical currents and chemical interactions. It's through this intricate web of cells that your body and brain communicate.

Two main components make up your nervous system: your central nervous system, which includes your brain and spinal cord, and your peripheral nervous system. Your peripheral nerves extend from your spinal cord to your skin, muscles and internal organs. Within each of these systems are three major categories of nerves:

- **Autonomic nerves.** They maintain normal body processes, such as heart rate, breathing, blood pressure, digestion, perspiration and sexual function.
- **Motor nerves.** They're responsible for movement of your muscles. Your motor nerves allow you to move your hands and feet, to walk or to sit.
- **Sensory nerves.** These are your sensing nerves. They allow you to feel an object when you touch it. They also allow you to feel pain.

The good news, though, is that despite having persistent pain, you can still enjoy an active, productive and satisfying lifestyle.

Managing chronic pain has evolved from a time when it was thought that pain was something to be tolerated and endured, and that complaining or seeking relief was a sign of weakness.

Research and experience have determined that pain is something that should be considered when evaluating the condition of a person seeking medical care. In fact, pain is sometimes referred to as the fifth vital sign, and doctors are urged to assess their patients for pain at the same time they check a patient's four main vital signs — pulse, blood pressure, body temperature and respiration.

The Joint Commission — formerly known as the Joint Commission on Accreditation of Healthcare Organizations (JCAHO) — sets and enforces standards of care in hospitals and other health care facilities. Understanding the important role pain plays in a person's health and recovery, the Joint Commission has developed a list of standards designed to ensure the assessment and treatment of pain for every patient.

The bottom line is, pain is common and complex. The purpose of this book is to help you better understand your pain and its harmful effects, and perhaps more importantly, to offer guidance on how you can take control of your pain — instead of letting it control you.

How you feel pain

Understanding the mechanism that causes your body to perceive pain can help you better appreciate why it is that you experience pain. It can also help you better understand why chronic pain is often difficult to treat.

Pain results from a series of electrical and chemical exchanges involving three major components: your peripheral nerves, spinal cord and brain.

Peripheral nerves

Your peripheral nerves encompass a network of nerve fibers that branches throughout your body. Attached to some of these fibers are special nerve endings that can sense an unpleasant stimulus, such as a cut, burn or painful pressure. These nerve endings are called nociceptors (no-sih-SEP-turs).

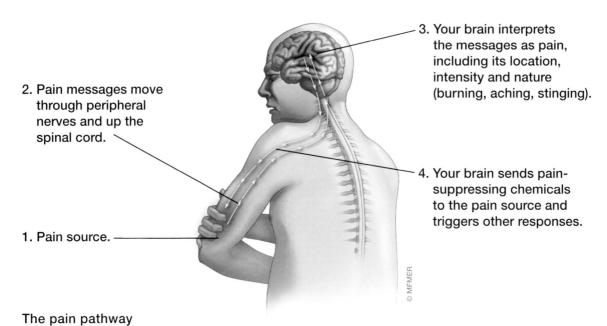

3. Your brain interprets the messages as pain, including its location, intensity and nature (burning, aching, stinging).

2. Pain messages move through peripheral nerves and up the spinal cord.

4. Your brain sends pain-suppressing chemicals to the pain source and triggers other responses.

1. Pain source.

© MFMER

The pain pathway

Pain results from a series of complex electrical and chemical changes involving your peripheral nerves, spinal cord and brain.

You have millions of nociceptors in your skin, bones, joints and muscles and in the protective membrane around your internal organs.

Nociceptors are concentrated in areas of your body more prone to injury, such as your fingers and toes. That's why a splinter in your finger hurts more than one in your back or shoulder. There may be as many as 1,300 nociceptors in just one square inch of skin. Muscles, protected beneath your skin, have fewer nerve endings. And internal organs, protected by skin, muscle and bone, have fewer still.

Some nociceptors sense sharp blows, others heat. One type senses pressure, temperature and chemical changes. Nociceptors can also detect inflammation caused by injury, disease or infection.

When nociceptors detect a harmful stimulus, they relay their pain messages in the form of electrical impulses along a peripheral nerve to your spinal cord and brain. However, the speed by which the messages travel can vary. Sensations of severe pain are transmitted almost instantaneously. Dull, aching pain — such as an upset stomach or an earache — is relayed on fibers that transmit at a slower speed.

Spinal cord

When pain messages reach your spinal cord, they meet up with specialized nerve cells that act as gatekeepers. The nerve cells filter the pain messages on their way to your brain.

For severe pain that's linked to bodily harm, such as when you touch a hot stove, the "gate" is wide open and the messages take an express route to your brain. Nerve cells in your spinal cord also respond to these urgent warnings by triggering other parts of the nervous system into action, such as your motor nerves. Your motor nerves signal your muscles to pull your hand away from the burner.

Weak pain messages, however, such as from a scratch, may receive a different response. They may be filtered or blocked by the gate.

Within your spinal cord, the messages can also change. Other sensations may overpower and diminish the pain signals, such as when you massage the injured area. The warnings sent by your peripheral nerves are downgraded to a lower priority. Nerve cells in your spinal cord may also release chemicals that amplify or diminish the messages, affecting the strength of the pain signal.

Brain

When pain messages reach your brain, they arrive at the thalamus, a sorting and switching station deep inside your brain. The thalamus interprets the messages as pain and forwards them simultaneously to three specialized regions: the physical sensation region (somatosensory cortex), the emotional and feeling region (limbic system), and the thinking region (frontal cortex). Your awareness of pain becomes a complex experience affected by these three regions.

Your brain responds to the pain messages by sending back messages that promote the healing process. For instance, if you've cut your finger, your brain signals your autonomic nervous system, the system that controls blood flow, to send additional blood and nutrients to the injury site. It also dispatches the release of pain-suppressing chemicals and sends stop-pain messages to the injury site.

Your pain response

When pain messages reach your brain, two things generally determine how you respond to them — the physical sensation associated with the messages and your individual characteristics.

Physical sensation

Pain results when pain receptors in your body become injured or inflamed due to an injury or illness. Pain comes in many forms: sharp, jabbing, throbbing, burning, stinging, tingling, nagging, dull and aching. It also varies from mild to severe. Severe pain grabs your attention quickly and often produces a greater physical and emotional response than does mild pain. Severe pain can also incapacitate you, making it difficult or impossible to sit or stand.

However, the physical sensation associated with pain is more than just the effects of tissue damage. Pain pathways that travel through your spinal cord also pass through a number of areas within your brain, affecting how you experience pain. As pain messages

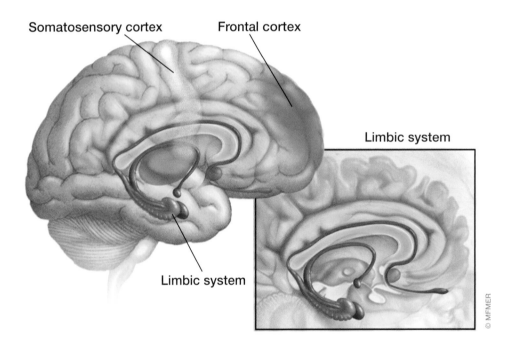

Your brain and pain

Three brain areas influence how you respond to pain. The somatosensory cortex deciphers the physical sensation — is the pain sharp and jabbing or dull and aching? The limbic system controls your emotional response — do you cry out in agony or disregard it as an annoyance? The frontal cortex governs your physical reaction, such as pulling your hand away from a hot burner or rubbing a bump on your head.

Natural painkillers and pain enhancers

Your brain and spinal cord produce their own painkillers, which are similar to the narcotic drug morphine, used to treat severe pain. Two types of morphine-like pain relievers are endorphins and enkephalins. When released, these substances attach to special receptors in your brain, producing stop-pain messages.

Other substances in your body do the opposite. They intensify your pain. A protein called substance P stimulates nerve endings at the injury site and within your spinal cord, increasing pain messages. Other pain enhancers work by activating normally silent nerve cells in the injured area. This activation prompts the cells to generate pain messages even when the stimulation they detect isn't painful. This not only worsens the pain but also enlarges the area of sensitivity.

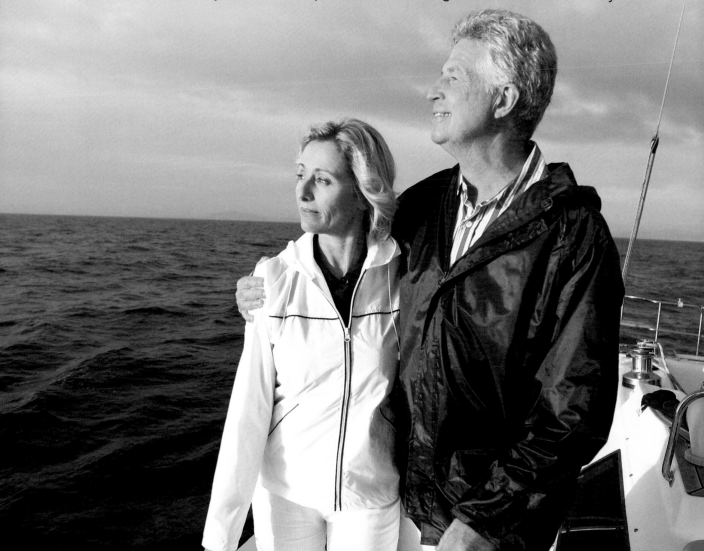

travel to the brain's emotional and feeling region (limbic system) and thinking region (frontal cortex), they may be altered by a number of factors such as anxiety, fear, past pain experiences and the pain experiences of loved ones.

Individuality

People respond to pain in different ways because pain is made up of many unique components. Equally important in the experience of pain is who you are. Your reaction to pain is heavily influenced by your personal traits and characteristics.

An injury or illness that may be painful for one person may only be slightly bothersome for another. Why is this? Many factors are thought to affect how you sense and react to pain. Your personal genetics, including how sensitive your body is to pain signals is a key component. Other factors that influence your response to pain include:

- How you naturally think, learn and reason
- Your expectations as to how you "think" you should feel
- How attentive you are to your body's responses — what your body seems to be telling you

- Whether you're dealing with other illnesses or conditions, such as depression or anxiety, that can affect how you sense and react to pain

In addition, memories of past painful experiences, cultural factors, and your upbringing and attitude also affect how you interpret pain messages and tolerate pain. For example, a minor sensation that would barely register as pain, such as a dentist's probe, can actually produce exaggerated pain for a child who's never been to the dentist and is nervous about it.

But your emotional state can also work in your favor. This was illustrated by a study that compared formerly wounded war veterans with men in the general population. Men in both groups had the same kind of surgery. The combat veterans, however, required less pain medication than the others did, perhaps because they thought that the surgery was a minor matter compared with what they'd experienced in battle.

So, pain literally is "in your head." There's no way to disentangle tissue damage due to injury or illness from the complex emotional and cognitive processing that accompanies the pain experience.

Acute pain vs. chronic pain

There are two major categories of pain. Acute pain is triggered by tissue damage and is designed to protect you from further injury. Acute pain is the type of pain that generally accompanies illness, injury or surgery. It may be mild and last just a moment, such as from an insect sting. Or it can be severe and last for weeks or months, such as from a burn, pulled muscle or broken bone.

With acute pain, you typically know exactly where it hurts — the term *acute* refers to severe or sudden pain. A toothache from a cavity, a burning elbow from a scrape and pain from a surgical incision are examples of acute pain. With time and treatment of the underlying cause, the pain generally fades away — when the cavity is filled, the skin grows back or the incision heals.

Chronic pain refers to persistent pain — pain that continues after the injury is healed. Pain is generally described as chronic when it lasts three months or longer. This is reflected in the word itself. Chronic comes from the Greek word for "time."

As with acute pain, chronic pain spans the full range of sensations and intensities. It can feel tingling, jolting, burning, dull or sharp. The pain may remain constant, or it may come and go, like a migraine that develops without warning.

Unlike acute pain, however, with chronic pain you may not know the reason for the pain. The original injury shows every indication of being healed, yet the pain remains — and it may be even more intense.

Chronic pain can also occur without any indication of an injury or illness. Years ago, people who complained of pain that had no apparent cause were thought to be imagining the misery or trying to get attention. Doctors now know this is not true. Chronic pain is real.

What causes chronic pain?

Frequently, the cause of chronic pain isn't well understood. There may be no evidence of disease or damage to your body tissues that doctors can directly link to the pain.

Sometimes, chronic pain is due to a chronic condition, such as arthritis, which produces painful inflammation in your joints; fibromyalgia, which causes aching in your muscles; or a migraine, which causes swelling of blood vessels in your brain and scalp.

Occasionally, chronic pain may stem from an accident, infection or surgery that damages a peripheral or spinal nerve. This type of nerve pain that lingers after the original injury heals is called neuropathic pain — meaning the damaged nerve, not the original injury, is causing the pain. Neuropathic pain can also result from diseases such as diabetes or alcoholism, which can damage the body's nerves.

Once damaged, a nerve may send pain messages that are unwarranted. For example, metabolic changes associated with diabetes can damage the small nerves in your hands and feet, producing a tingling and painful burning sensation.

Little is known about why injured nerves sometimes misfire and send painful messages. However, one reason is that when a nerve is destroyed, the severed end can sprout a tangle of disorganized nerve fibers (neuroma). This bundle of nerve tissue then starts sending spontaneous pain signals. These fibers also refuse to follow normal checks and balances that keep pain at bay.

Sensitization

Scientific research continues to provide new knowledge of how pain is transmitted and how the experience of pain is created in the brain.

One important aspect of these discoveries about pain has to do with a process called sensitization. An introduction to sensitization can help you to understand why it is that chronic pain can be so severe and why your pain may seem out of proportion to the type of injury or disease that you experienced.

The intricate biology involved in sensitization is complex, but the basic idea behind it is fairly straightforward. When pain signals are transmitted from injured or diseased tissues to the brain, during their transmission the signals may activate (sensitize) pain circuits in other locations of the body, such as the peripheral nerves and spinal cord.

The process of sensitization can be compared to the volume control on your stereo, amplifying — and sometimes distorting — the pain message. The result is a painful condition that's severe and out of proportion to the disease or original injury.

Sensitization may affect all regions of your nervous system that process pain messages, including the sensing, feeling and thinking centers of the brain. When this occurs, chronic pain also may be associated with emotional and psychological suffering.

An example of sensitization is phantom limb pain. In this condition, a person can feel intense pain in the location of a missing body part, for example, pain in an arm or a leg that's been amputated and is no longer there. Phantom limb pain, which is difficult to treat, is explained by persistent activation (sensitization) of the pain transmission pathways. The injured limb is no longer there, but the pathways in which pain messages were transmitted are acting as if it still were.

Considerable scientific research around the world is focused on identifying the molecular and cellular processes that are involved in sensitization. The results of this research are likely to provide new and better treatments for many types of chronic pain.

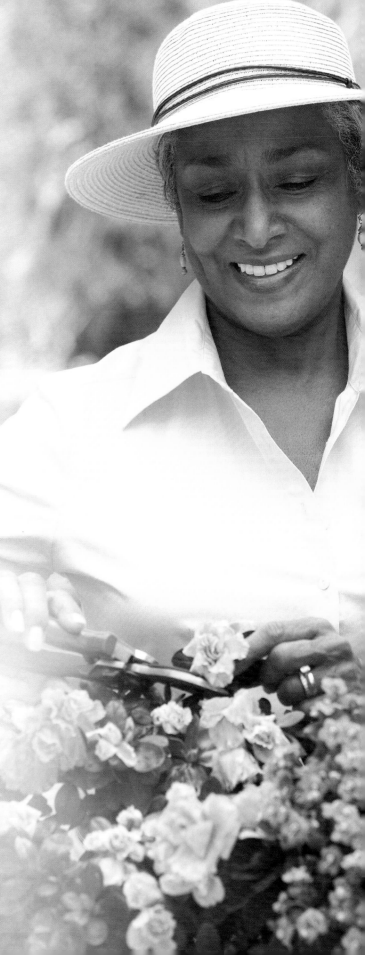

Chronic pain challenges

Because pain is such a personal experience, persistent pain can be difficult to treat. Occasionally, surgery can cure or reduce pain. And for some types of chronic pain, medication or injections are beneficial. Frequently, though, none of these approaches is very effective by themselves.

But that doesn't mean there isn't any hope. You may not be able to take a pill to make your pain disappear, but you can learn how to manage your pain and improve your quality of life.

Living well despite chronic pain has a lot to do with your attitude and your lifestyle. If you have a negative attitude and view yourself as a victim of your pain, the pain will continue to control you and consume your energy. On the other hand, if you approach your condition with a positive attitude and a willingness to change, you're likely to be successful in coping with your pain.

In the chapters that follow, we provide key steps to help you live better with chronic pain. Not only can this book help you discover what may be contributing to your pain, it also includes strategies and suggestions for how to make positive life changes. With your doctor, other health care professionals, and your family and friends, you can learn to take control of your pain — and your life.

Chapter 3

Common types of chronic pain

Chronic pain can affect just about any part of your body, from your head to your toes, from your skin to your internal organs. Your pain may be related to an existing illness or stem from an accident or injury. Perhaps your pain is linked to a condition that doctors don't fully understand. Or maybe it has no apparent cause.

Arthritis pain, back pain and headache are the most common types of chronic pain, but many other conditions can produce persistent pain. In this chapter, we discuss some of the more common disorders and diseases that can lead to chronic pain and the culprit behind the pain. Knowing what's triggering the pain is helpful. There are times, though, when a cause can't be found. This doesn't mean the pain isn't real, it just may be more difficult to treat.

Arthritis

The term *arthritis* means joint inflammation. Although people often talk about it as one disease, it's not. There are many forms of arthritis. Some forms begin gradually. Others appear suddenly and then disappear, only to return again later.

Arthritis can affect any joint in your body, and it may be triggered by various causes, including an injury, lack of physical activity, natural wear on your joints or genetic disease. Depending on the type of arthritis you have, your signs and symptoms may include pain, stiffness, swelling, redness and decreased range of motion. The two most common forms of arthritis are osteoarthritis and rheumatoid arthritis.

Normal spine

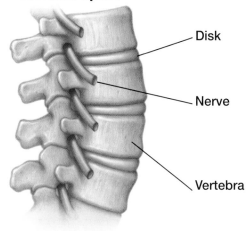

- Disk
- Nerve
- Vertebra

Spine with osteoarthritis

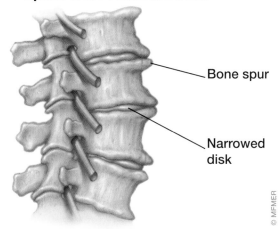

- Bone spur
- Narrowed disk

© MFMER

Osteoarthritis

Elastic structures called disks serve as cushions between vertebrae in a normal spine, keeping it flexible. In osteoarthritis, disks narrow, leading to bony lumps along the edges of vertebrae, called spurs. Pain and stiffness may occur where bone surfaces rub together.

Osteoarthritis

About half of all people with arthritis have osteoarthritis, which affects approximately 27 million Americans. This condition results when cartilage that cushions the ends of bones in your joints deteriorates. If the cartilage wears down completely, you may be left with bone rubbing against bone, irritating the joint and producing pain.

Your body tries to repair the damage, but often the repairs are unsuccessful, resulting in growth of new bone along the sides of existing bone. The new

bone may produce bony lumps, most noticeably in your hands and feet, especially in the joints of your fingers and toes. These lumps, called spurs, may or may not produce pain and tenderness.

Osteoarthritis most often develops after age 45 and occurs equally in men and women. It can develop anywhere in your body, but it tends to be most common in your hands and feet, neck, lower back, knees, and hips. The disease generally results from wear on your joints or a joint injury. It may also stem from an imbalance of enzymes in a joint, causing cartilage to break down.

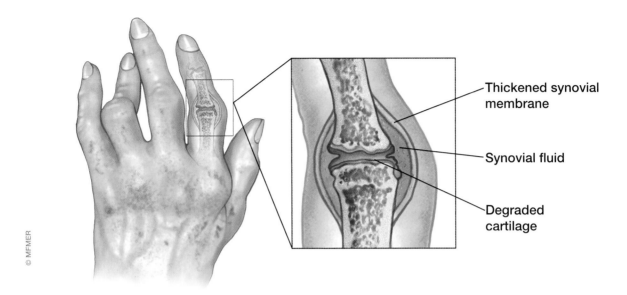

Thickened synovial membrane

Synovial fluid

Degraded cartilage

Rheumatoid arthritis

Rheumatoid arthritis often leads to deformity of the fingers and hands. During flare-ups of the disease, your hands may be painful and weak.

Initially, the pain may be minor and hurt only when you use the affected joint. In time, it can intensify and hurt even when you're not using the joint.

Rheumatoid arthritis

Unlike osteoarthritis, rheumatoid arthritis is thought to stem from an immune system disorder that causes your immune system to attack the lining in your joints. White blood cells move into joint tissues, producing inflammation and pain. Swelling of the tissues triggers the release of natural chemicals that damage cartilage, tendons and ligaments. Gradually, the joint loses its shape and may be destroyed.

Rheumatoid arthritis most often affects joints in your wrists, hands, feet and ankles. It can also affect your elbows, shoulders, hips, knees, neck and jaw. In addition to pain and swelling, you may experience stiffness and loss of motion in the joints.

The disease typically develops between ages 20 and 50. An estimated 1.3 million Americans have rheumatoid arthritis, and roughly twice as many women as men are affected by it.

Back pain

Most adults experience at least one bout of back pain during their lifetimes. And millions of Americans have back pain on a frequent basis. In fact, back pain is one of the most common reasons for health care visits and missed work.

Most back pain occurs in your lower back (lumbar area), which bears most of your weight. Your lower back also serves as your body's pivot point, allowing you to bend forward and backward and twist sideways.

Acute back pain often stems from an injury or overuse. Usually, there's an accumulation of stress with one particular event causing the pain. Sometimes, though, back pain can occur for no specific reason and frequently recur. This is often referred to as chronic nonspecific back pain. What causes some people to experience this type of pain isn't always clear. Oftentimes, back pain is related to one of the following conditions.

Muscle strain and spasm

Muscle strain is a common cause of back pain — especially pain that occurs in the lower back. Muscle strain can result if you lift something too heavy, twist too sharply or stand on your feet too long. Excess body weight and poor posture also can lead to muscle strain. When your back muscles become strained, they also can spasm, or "knot up."

Spasm is your back's response to injury, designed to immobilize you and prevent further damage. Any movement of the injured muscles can set off a wave of stabbing pains.

The good news is the vast majority of these strains resolve within a few weeks, usually about two weeks. But in a small percentage of people, healing can take longer. In some cases, the pain never goes away and becomes a chronic problem.

Sciatica

This condition is named for the large nerve known as the sciatic nerve that extends down each leg from your buttock to your heel. Inflammation or compression of a nerve root in your lower back can cause sciatica. You may feel the pain radiating from your back down through your buttock to your lower leg. Tingling, numbness or muscle weakness also may occur.

Another cause of sciatica is related to spasms or tightness in the buttock (gluteal) muscles. This is called piriformis syndrome.

Usually, the pain goes away on its own. However, severe nerve compression can cause progressive muscle weakness and continued pain.

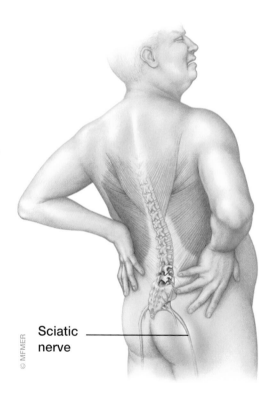

Sciatic nerve

Sciatica

Sciatica is pain that radiates from your back down through your buttock to your lower leg. It may be caused by inflammation or compression of spinal nerve roots that merge to form your sciatic nerve.

Herniated disk

Injury or normal wear and tear can cause a disk between the bones in your back (vertebrae) to bulge or rupture. This is sometimes called a slipped disk. When the disk ruptures, the rubber-like interior of the disk pokes out from its normal position between your vertebrae.

Almost everyone older than age 40 has one or more bulging disks, and most people aren't bothered by them. But if the bulging material presses against an adjacent nerve, the condition can produce pain. Generally, the rupture heals over time and the pain goes away. But in some cases, nerve compression and pain can persist.

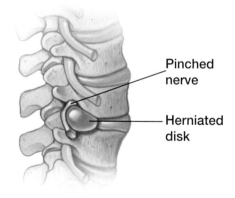

Pinched nerve

Herniated disk

Herniated disk

Wear and tear or injury can cause disks to rupture (herniate), creating painful pressure on nerves.

Additional causes

Other conditions that may lead to chronic back pain include:

- Joint degeneration from arthritis
- Reduced muscle tone caused by physical inactivity

Complex regional pain syndrome

Complex regional pain syndrome is an uncommon form of chronic pain that usually affects an arm or leg. A minor injury can set off this painful condition. So can a stroke or heart attack. Before long, you're experiencing a variety of painful symptoms, not only at the injury site but also in adjacent locations — and the pain is out of proportion to the severity of the initial injury.

Many cases of complex regional pain syndrome occur after a forceful trauma, such as a crush injury, fracture or amputation. Other major and minor traumas — such as surgery, infections and even sprained ankles — can lead to complex regional pain syndrome. Emotional stress may be a precipitating factor, as well.

It's not well understood why these injuries can trigger complex regional pain syndrome, but it may be due to a dysfunctional interaction between your central nervous and peripheral nervous systems and inappropriate inflammatory responses. There are two types of complex regional pain syndrome.

Type 1. Previously known as reflex sympathetic dystrophy, this type occurs after an illness or injury that didn't directly damage the nerves in your affected limb. About 90 percent of people with complex regional pain syndrome have type 1.

Type 2. Once referred to as causalgia, this type follows a distinct nerve injury.

Complex regional pain syndrome is difficult to diagnose because it's similar to other conditions. However, it typically includes these unique characteristics:

- Pain that lasts longer and is more intense than you would expect from the injury
- Blood flow changes that alter the temperature, color and thickness of skin in the affected area
- Persistent swelling of the affected area

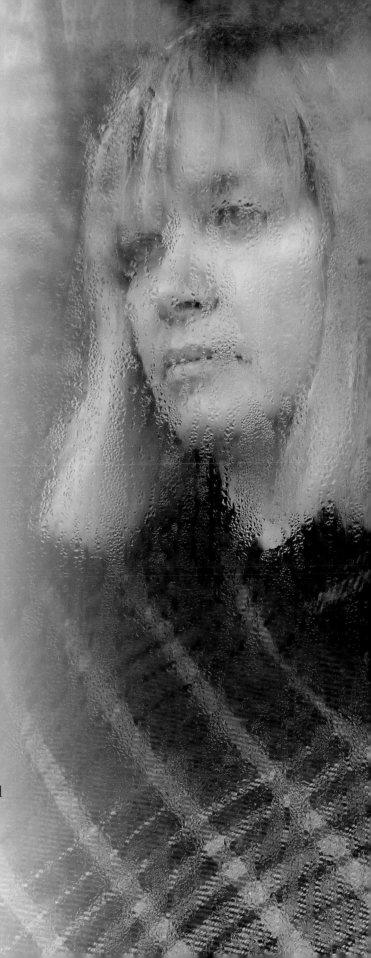

In some people, the signs and symptoms eventually go away on their own. In others, they may persist for months to years.

Fibromyalgia

Fibromyalgia is a collection of symptoms that includes chronic widespread pain with tenderness, fatigue, sleep difficulties and anxiety. It may coexist with other diseases and disorders such as osteoarthritis, rheumatoid arthritis, and neurological conditions such as multiple sclerosis.

The main symptom of fibromyalgia is pain and tenderness throughout the body accompanied by an overwhelming sense of fatigue. The pain may be a deep ache or a burning sensation. Other signs and symptoms associated with fibromyalgia may include:

- Digestive problems
- Difficulty sleeping
- Numbness
- Stiffness
- Tingling
- Headache
- Sensitivity to medications, food, and weather and temperature changes
- Pain during menstruation

- Dizziness
- Mood changes

Because these signs and symptoms commonly occur together and no specific cause has been found, fibromyalgia is referred to as a syndrome rather than a disease. In addition, because the symptoms are many and varied and don't follow a consistent pattern, fibromyalgia can be stressful as well as painful.

Most often, symptoms of fibromyalgia first become noticeable in your 30s. They may flare up and then subside, but they usually don't disappear completely. Although fibromyalgia tends to stay with you, it isn't progressive or life-threatening.

It's likely that a number of factors contribute to the development of fibromyalgia. One theory, called central sensitization, holds that people with fibromyalgia may have a lower threshold for pain because of increased sensitivity in the brain to pain signals. Other factors may include release of inflammatory substances called cytokines, sleep deprivation from untreated sleep disorders, injury, sympathetic nervous system abnormalities, medications, food and changes in muscle metabolism.

A recent Mayo Clinic study found that many people with fibromyalgia — especially men — go undiagnosed. Results indicated that 20 times more men appeared to have fibromyalgia than had been diagnosed with the condition, while three times more women reported fibromyalgia symptoms than were diagnosed.

Headache

Of all the pains people experience, headache is a common complaint. Nearly everyone gets a headache at some point. Headaches can range from fleeting annoyances to those that lay you flat on your back and return often enough they become a chronic problem. There are several types of headaches. Most fall into one of two categories.

Tension-type

This is the most common type of headache. It can range from mild to severe and can disrupt your daily routine to varying degrees. You may experience dull, tight, pressurized or throbbing pain that envelopes your forehead, scalp, the back of the neck or both sides of your head.

Tension-type headaches may be triggered by stressful events such as a demanding job, a bumper-to-bumper commute, or an argument with a friend or family member. Staring at a computer screen all day or other prolonged, stressful postures also can produce tension-type headaches. These headaches can become a chronic problem.

Migraine

More than 20 percent of women and about 10 percent of men experience a more painful variety of headache known as a migraine. This type of headache not only gets your attention, but can put your life on hold.

Migraines generally produce a throbbing pain on one side of your head — often your temple or forehead. Lights and loud noises may intensify the pain, and you may become nauseated and vomit. The pain can range from moderate to severe. Most migraines occur for only a few hours before peaking and slowly subsiding.

Migraines may be caused by changes in the brainstem and its interactions with the trigeminal nerve, a major pain pathway. Imbalances in brain chemicals — including serotonin, which helps regulate pain in your nervous system — also may be involved. Researchers continue to study the role of serotonin in migraines.

Approximately 25 percent of people with recurrent migraines get warnings of an impending headache. These signals, called auras, may involve tingling sensations or visual distortions, such as blurred vision or zigzagging lights. They generally last less than an hour.

Migraines are thought to be hereditary, but they may be triggered by a number of different factors.

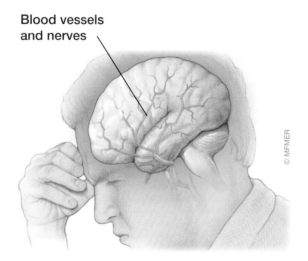

Blood vessels and nerves

© MFMER

Migraine

A migraine appears to stem from an imbalance of brain chemicals that causes blood vessels in your brain to swell and signal pain.

Hormone fluctuations. Three times more women than men are affected by migraines. In a number of women, their headaches occur only during menstruation or right beforehand. Some women experience migraines throughout their cycle, but the headaches worsen right before their period. Estrogen found in birth control pills and in hormone therapy also may trigger migraine attacks in some women. For other women, their migraines diminish when taking estrogen.

Diet. Some people with migraines point to a particular food as a trigger for their attacks. The foods vary but the most common culprits tend to be alcohol — especially red wine and beer — aged cheeses, chocolate, caffeine, monosodium glutamate (MSG), and fermented, pickled or marinated foods. Going too long without eating and caffeine withdrawal also can cause migraines.

Environment. Many people cite bright lights, strong odors or changes in weather conditions as triggers for their migraines.

Lifestyle. Daily stress can trigger a migraine. Migraines may also result from poor or changing sleep patterns, extreme fatigue and stress, as well as relief from stress. It's not uncommon for a migraine to occur on a quiet Saturday after a very stressful week.

Medications. Several medications may trigger or aggravate a migraine in people who are susceptible to such headaches. These medications include certain high blood pressure drugs, birth control pills and hormone therapy. Frequent use of pain medication, including over-the-counter pain relievers, also may trigger a headache when the dose wears off. This is called a rebound withdrawal (medication-overuse) headache.

Irritable bowel syndrome

Irritable bowel syndrome (IBS) is a complex disorder of the lower intestinal tract that causes pain, bloating, gas, and recurrent bouts of diarrhea or constipation. It's a common gastrointestinal disorder and a frequent reason people see a doctor. Fortunately, IBS doesn't cause inflammation or structural damage.

The pain accompanying this condition often occurs below the navel and may be dull and aching or sharp and sudden.

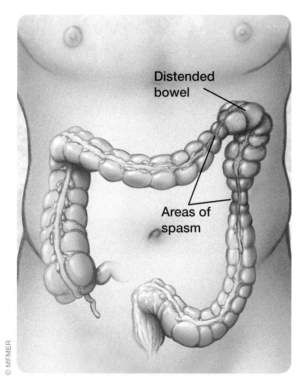

Irritable bowel syndrome

A spasm in the bowel wall may cause abdominal pain and other unpleasant symptoms commonly associated with irritable bowel syndrome.

The condition may stem from disturbances in the nerves that control sensation or from muscle contractions in your bowel. Your central nervous system or hormonal changes also may play a role. Hormone fluctuations help explain why some women's symptoms are worse before or during menstruation.

Some evidence suggests that people with IBS have intestines that react more strongly to factors such as stress,

activity or diet than do those in people without the condition. There's little evidence that IBS results from particular foods. However, in some cases, fatty foods, beans and other gas-producing foods, alcohol, caffeine, and high-fiber foods may worsen symptoms.

Like many people, you may have only mild signs and symptoms of irritable bowel syndrome. Sometimes, though, the condition can be disabling. For most people, IBS is a chronic condition, with times when the signs and symptoms are worse and times when they improve or even disappear completely.

Mouth, jaw and face pain

Some people experience chronic pain in the mouth, jaws and face (orofacial pain). Often, this pain is the result of dental problems, such as cavities or gum disease. But sometimes it can stem from other orofacial conditions.

Burning mouth syndrome

With burning mouth syndrome, you may have a burning sensation on your

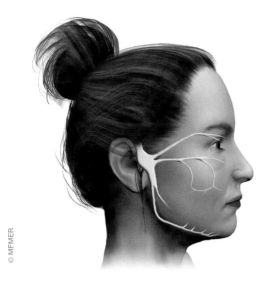

© MFMER

Trigeminal neuralgia

If you have trigeminal neuralgia, pain may occur in areas supplied by one of the three branches of the trigeminal (fifth cranial) nerve.

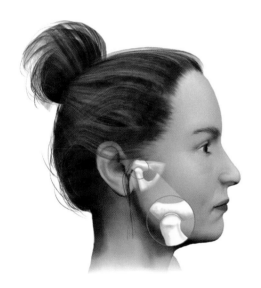

Temporomandibular joint

Your temporomandibular joint is where the lower jawbone connects with the skull's temporal bone. Inflammation, injury or dislocation of the joint may cause pain.

tongue or lips, or more widespread burning that involves your entire mouth. Burning mouth syndrome affects women seven times as often as men. It generally occurs in middle-aged or older adults. Possible causes of the condition include chronic infections, reflux of stomach acid, blood diseases, hormone imbalances and side effects of some medications. However, for many people the cause of burning mouth syndrome is unknown.

Trigeminal neuralgia

Also known as tic douloureux (doo-loo-ROO), this form of pain can develop when a blood vessel comes in contact with the trigeminal nerve, putting pressure on the nerve. The trigeminal nerve branches throughout your face and controls facial sensations and some muscles involved in chewing.

Trigeminal neuralgia can cause an electric shock-like pain on one side of your face and may cause you to wince as if you've been hit in the face. Jolts of pain may persist from a few seconds to a minute or two, usually returning many times a day.

Most trigeminal neuralgia pain occurs spontaneously, but the pain sometimes may be triggered by touching your face, eating, talking or brushing your teeth. Even the feeling of a breeze on your face can trigger the pain.

Temporomandibular joint disorders

The temporomandibular joints, located on each side of your face, connect your jaw to your skull. Temporomandibular joint disorders refers to a group of symptoms affecting these joints and their attached muscles.

A common symptom is pain in your jaw, face, neck or ear. Other signs and symptoms may include headaches, jaw locking or catching, and pops or clicks in your jaw during normal use.

There are several theories as to the causes of these disorders. They include trauma to the joints, degeneration of the joints and disturbance of the muscles surrounding the joints.

Other causes

Orofacial pain can also occur for other reasons that aren't well understood.

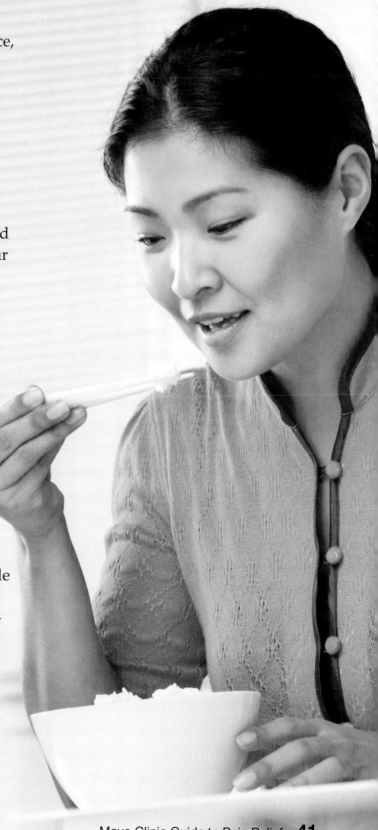

Many times, the pain develops after dental treatment or a facial injury. It may be a constant aching or burning. Or it may come in the form of frequent shocks. Nerve damage in a tooth and damage to nerves in your face are possible causes. Postherpetic neuralgia (see page 47) also can cause facial pain.

Neck pain

An injury, repetitive motions or poor posture that lead to fatigue and overuse can strain the muscles, ligaments or tendons in your neck, producing inflammation and pain. Poor posture — whether it's leaning into your computer at work or hunching over your workbench at home — is a common cause of neck pain. Most of the time the pain lasts for just a few days or weeks. Occasionally, though, the pain can become chronic.

Neck pain may also stem from a herniated disk or degeneration of joints in your upper spine due to osteoarthritis. Instead of sliding across each other smoothly, bony surfaces in your neck grate on each other, producing pain.

In addition, with age, the disks that cushion the vertebrae in your spinal

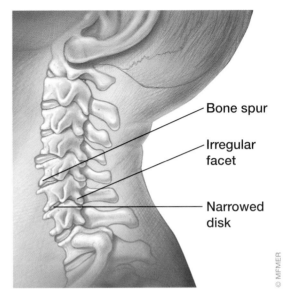

Neck pain

Disks between bones in your neck can thin and lose elasticity. Bony outgrowths (spurs) may form. As joints rub together, surfaces where they meet become irregular and pain may result.

column can become dry. When this occurs, the spaces in your spine where the nerves exit become narrowed and adjacent nerves become irritated. Other tissues and bony growths also can press on your nerves as they exit your spinal cord, causing pain.

Often, one pain leads to another. For example, when you feel pain from an injury or arthritis, you automatically tense your neck muscles to prevent movement in the sore spot. The tension in your neck also produces pain and can trigger a painful muscle spasm.

Overuse strain injuries

These injuries result from overuse of your muscles and tendons — mainly those in your hands, wrists and arms. The most noticeable symptom is pain. But an overuse injury can also cause tingling, weakness, numbness, swelling and stiffness.

Computer users, meat cutters, assembly line employees and athletes are among those commonly affected by an overuse injury. But this type of injury can occur in anyone who regularly uses repeated motions of the hands, wrists and shoulders while performing daily activities.

Carpal tunnel syndrome is the most recognized overuse injury. It results from constant strain on your wrist, which can inflame the tendons located below your carpal ligament, the ligament that stretches across the palm side of your wrist.

As the tendons become inflamed and swollen, they press against a nearby nerve also located beneath the carpal ligament. Pressure on this nerve is what produces the pain associated with carpal tunnel syndrome. Because the

nerve runs up your arm all the way to your neck, you might feel pain anywhere along that pathway.

Most often, the result is intermittent numbness, tingling or pain that starts in your wrist and moves down into your thumb and first two or three

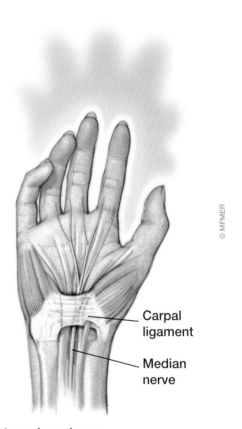

© MFMER

Carpal ligament

Median nerve

Carpal tunnel syndrome
A narrow tunnel through your wrist (the carpal tunnel) protects your median nerve, which provides sensation to your fingers. When swelling occurs in the tunnel, the median nerve can become compressed, producing pain.

What is phantom pain?

Phantom pain is pain that feels like it's coming from a body part that's no longer there. Doctors once believed this post-amputation phenomenon was a psychological problem, but experts now recognize that these real sensations originate in the spinal cord and brain.

Although phantom pain occurs most often in people who've had an arm or leg removed, the disorder may also occur after surgeries to remove other body parts, such as a breast or eye or the penis or tongue.

For some people, phantom pain gets better over time without treatment. For others, managing phantom pain can be challenging. You and your doctor can work together to treat phantom pain effectively with medication or other therapies.

Symptoms

Most people who've had a limb removed report that it sometimes feels as if their amputated limb is still there. This painless phenomenon, known as phantom limb sensation, can also occur in people who were born without limbs. Phantom limb sensations may include feelings of coldness, warmth, or itchiness or tingling — but should not be confused with phantom pain. Similarly, pain from the remaining stump of an amputated limb is not phantom pain. By definition, phantom pain feels as if it comes from a body part that no longer remains.

Characteristics of phantom pain include:

- Onset within the first few days of amputation
- Tendency to come and go rather than be constant
- Usually affects the part of the limb farthest from the body, such as the foot of an amputated leg
- Described as shooting, stabbing, boring, squeezing, throbbing or burning
- May feel as if the phantom part is forced into an uncomfortable position
- May be triggered by weather changes, pressure on the remaining part of the limb or emotional stress

Causes

The exact cause of phantom pain is unclear, but it appears to originate in the spinal cord and brain. During imaging scans — such as magnetic resonance imaging (MRI) or positron emission tomography (PET) — portions of the brain that had been neurologically connected to the nerves of the amputated limb show activity when the person feels phantom pain.

Many experts believe phantom pain may be at least partially explained as a response to mixed signals from the brain. After an amputation, areas of the spinal cord and brain lose input from the missing limb and adjust to this detachment in unpredictable ways. Studies also show that, after an amputation, the brain may remap that part of the body's sensory circuitry to another part of the body. Because the amputated area is no longer able to receive sensory information, the information is referred elsewhere — from a missing hand to a still-present cheek, for example. So when the cheek is touched, it's as though the missing hand also is being touched. Because this is yet another version of tangled sensory wires, the result can be pain.

A number of other factors are believed to contribute to phantom pain, including damaged nerve endings and scar tissue at the site of the amputation.

Risk factors

It's still unknown why some people develop phantom pain after an amputation while others don't. Some factors that may increase your risk of phantom pain include:

- **Pain before amputation.** Some researchers have found that people who had pain in a limb before amputation are likely to have it afterward.
- **Stump pain.** People who have persistent stump pain usually have phantom pain, too. Stump pain can be caused by an abnormal growth on damaged nerve endings (neuroma) that often results in painful nerve activity.
- **Poor-fitting artificial limb (prosthesis).** If you think your artificial limb may not fit properly, or is causing pain, talk to your doctor.

fingers. Some people find their symptoms are worse at night because of the position of their wrist or arm while sleeping. Holding a book or driving a car also may trigger symptoms.

Pelvic pain

About 15 percent of women see a doctor for some form of chronic pelvic pain. No physical cause may be found for such pain, but here are some conditions associated with pelvic pain:

- Endometriosis results when cells from the lining of a woman's uterus (endometrium) migrate into the abdominal cavity and plant themselves on pelvic walls and the surfaces of the ovaries. Some women experience pain, often described as a pressure-like aching in the lower abdomen, that can be chronic.
- Pelvic floor tension myalgia is due to spasms of the pelvic floor muscles, which loop around the rectum and attach to the front of the pelvis.
- Chronic pelvic inflammatory disease may occur when a long-term infection causes the fallopian tubes to scar and stick to the ovaries.
- Interstitial cystitis is a bladder condition that affects mainly women. It results from chronic inflammation of the bladder wall. Symptoms generally include pressure, pain and tenderness around the bladder.
- Pelvic congestion syndrome may be caused by varicose-type veins in the pelvic area that may lead to blood pooling in the ovaries and pelvis.
- Ovarian remnant syndrome occurs when small pieces of ovary left behind after a hysterectomy become tiny, painful cysts.
- Fibroids are noncancerous uterine growths that rarely cause pain. But they can cause pressure or a feeling of heaviness in your lower abdomen.

Peripheral neuropathy

This nerve-related condition most often affects your hands and feet, causing a tingling pain that may be accompanied by numbness. In some cases, the pain may also be shooting or burning.

Peripheral neuropathy can result from many causes, such as the side effects of medication — including some chemotherapy drugs — as well as infection or vitamin deficiencies. The most common causes of peripheral neuropathy, however, are diabetes, alcoholism, autoimmune diseases such as rheumatoid arthritis or lupus, and hereditary neuropathies. There are also times when the cause is unclear.

The condition usually starts with a tingling sensation in your toes or the balls of your feet that spreads upward. Occasionally, it may begin in your hands and extend up your arms. Numbness and weakness may follow. Your skin also may become highly sensitive.

Peripheral neuropathy symptoms may improve with time, especially if the condition is caused by an underlying condition that can be treated.

Postherpetic neuralgia

Postherpetic neuralgia is a complication of shingles, which is caused by the chickenpox (herpes zoster) virus. Most cases of shingles clear up within a few weeks. When the pain lasts after the shingles rash and blisters have disappeared, it's called postherpetic neuralgia.

Postherpetic neuralgia affects your nerve fibers and skin, and the pain associated with postherpetic neuralgia can be severe enough to interfere with sleep and appetite. Damaged nerve fibers aren't able to send normal pain messages. Instead, the messages become distorted and exaggerated, producing unrelenting, often severe, pain.

The risk of postherpetic neuralgia increases with age, primarily affecting people older than 60. The area affected also makes a difference. When shingles occurs on the face, for example, the likelihood of postherpetic neuralgia is significantly higher than for other parts of the body.

There's no cure for postherpetic neuralgia, but there are treatments to help ease symptoms. For most people, postherpetic neuralgia improves over time.

Unknown causes

Sometimes, chronic pain develops for no apparent reason. Your doctor isn't able to link it to an identifiable physical cause or condition. This doesn't mean that the pain is imagined. It simply means that your pain may be associated with factors that are difficult to diagnose, or it may be due to physical processes not yet understood.

Your health is also affected by the interaction of your mind and body. For some people, psychological issues can play a role in chronic pain. For example, people who've endured sexual abuse or other kinds of physical abuse appear to have a greater risk of developing chronic pelvic or abdominal pain. It's unknown whether the pain is the result of physical injuries or if it stems from emotional scars or stress. It may be due to a combination of factors.

Chapter 4

Chronic pain cycles

People living with chronic pain often compare their lives to a roller coaster ride. There are good days when they feel uplifted and in control, followed by bad days when their mood sinks and they feel helpless. Rarely does pain stay at an even level; it fluctuates. Pain also doesn't have any boundaries. When a part of you is in pain, your whole body reacts.

As you try to understand, accept and manage your condition, your behavior and emotions may go through a series of ups and downs. This is especially true if you have debilitating pain — pain that prevents you from taking part in daily activities. The behavioral and emotional changes often associated with persistent pain tend to follow a predictable pattern. Similar to an experience of grief or deep sadness, you may move from one stage to the next.

Behavioral cycle

One of the first noticeable effects of chronic pain is the change it brings to your regular routine. Daily tasks often become more difficult to perform, or even impossible. Here is an example of how chronic pain can easily alter your routine and behavior.

Stage 1: Decrease in activity

Because of your pain, just getting the yard rake down from its hook in the garage — much less raking the entire yard — may seem like too big of a

Behavioral cycle

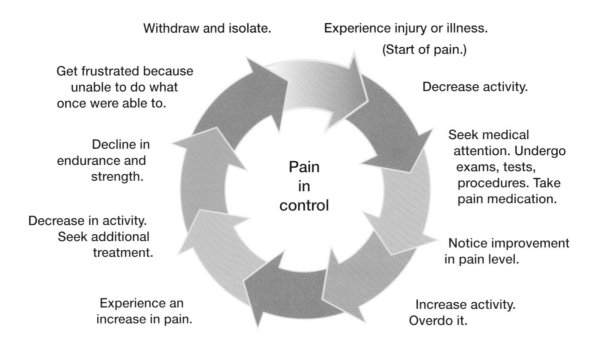

Experience injury or illness. (Start of pain.)

Decrease activity.

Seek medical attention. Undergo exams, tests, procedures. Take pain medication.

Notice improvement in pain level.

Increase activity. Overdo it.

Experience an increase in pain.

Decrease in activity. Seek additional treatment.

Decline in endurance and strength.

Get frustrated because unable to do what once were able to.

Withdraw and isolate.

Pain in control

Uncontrolled chronic pain commonly causes this pattern of behavior, beginning at the top of the circle and moving clockwise.

chore. So instead, you let the leaves fall. But every time you pass by a window, you're reminded of what you can't do.

There are other options: You could hire someone to rake the yard, but that would cost money. You could have your family do it, but you worry they'll feel resentful that you're not helping them. Plus, face it, you don't like watching others take over your responsibilities. So you decide to wait for a day when you feel better and you're up for the task.

Stage 2: Increase in activity

Finally, the day arrives when the pain is better, so you rake the yard. But you don't stop there. After what seemed like too much time on the couch, you decide to make up for lost hours. You run errands, clean the garage and go out to dinner with friends. On your feet all day long, you put in a day best fit for a superhero! But, hey, as long as you're feeling well, why not catch up on the things that you've been neglecting, right?

Communicating your pain

When you're in pain, others can often tell it by your actions. These actions, called pain behaviors, refer to things that you do or say that let people know you're in pain. Pain behaviors are ways of calling attention to your pain — either consciously or unconsciously.

Pain behaviors are a natural response to pain. Initially, especially for acute pain, they may help reduce your pain. But over time they become ineffective. For people with chronic pain, pain behaviors often become a habit. Some common pain behaviors include:

- Limping
- Staying in bed
- Crying
- Using protective posture
- Groaning

- Talking about pain, surgery or bodily functions
- Grimacing
- Limiting activity
- Withdrawing from others

People around you generally react in one of two ways to pain behaviors: They become annoyed by them — "Not this again" — or they become overly attentive to the behaviors — "Here, let me do that." Either response creates a situation in which people tend to focus more on your illness than on you. Pain behaviors also consume a lot of energy that could be channeled into more productive ventures, such as taking steps to manage your pain.

Stage 3: More pain, less activity

The next day, you can hardly move. You feel worse than you did before your superheroic day. You chastise yourself for trying to do too much and spend days resting and trying to recuperate.

Eventually, you begin to feel better. But as you become more active, your pain worsens. Thinking that the only way to control your pain is to limit all physical activity, you turn over your daily chores to family and friends and spend more time in bed or on the couch.

Meanwhile, more leaves fall, friends keep calling, and you don't feel up to doing anything.

Stage 4: Loss of strength and physical deconditioning

The time you spend lying around is making you tired, weak and less able to finish up the yardwork. Because of your long stretch of inactivity, your stamina is leaving you. You get fatigued easily. Even the thought of physical labor is daunting.

Stage 5: Withdrawal and isolation

You find yourself spending more time alone and less time with those who care about you. Because you've stopped going out with your friends, they've stopped calling. They figure that you'd just turn them down anyway, so why even bother?

Your family has gradually become accustomed to doing things without you. They now rake the yard without your help, and they've also started going out to dinner and attending social events without you. They think they're accommodating you by not forcing you to go.

In response, you find yourself retreating even further from your family, friends and favorite activities.

Eventually, a day comes when you begin to feel a little better. It's followed by another good day, and you become optimistic that your condition may finally be improving and before long you'll be back to your old self. But once again, your pain flares, and the cycle repeats itself.

Emotional cycle

Just as your behavior fluctuates when you're in pain, so do your emotions. Often, the two go hand in hand — the more you're able to do, the better your mood, and the less you're able to do, the worse your mood. Like your behaviors, your emotions also tend to follow a cyclic pattern.

Stage 1: Fear and concern

When you first begin to experience pain, you're fearful and concerned. You worry it may be a symptom of a serious disease. The more you worry, the worse it gets and the harder it becomes to ignore.

Stage 2: Hope and promise

When you finally learn what's triggering your pain, your fear and concern are replaced with hope that your doctor will be able to make the pain disappear and your life will soon return to normal. If your doctor isn't able to find a cause, at least knowing that your pain isn't a symptom of a life-threatening condition makes you feel better.

You think that curing your pain is a reasonable request. In today's society, when something breaks we expect someone to fix it. But repairing your body is far more complicated than fixing your car or a household appliance. When the pain continues to linger despite repeated trips to various doctors, your hope starts to diminish.

As you begin to realize that there may not be an answer to your problem, you may turn to easy fixes — behaviors and actions that provide temporary relief but have destructive consequences. This may include increasing your pain medication, drinking too much alcohol or using illicit drugs. These actions are

Overachiever's curse

Living with chronic pain isn't easy for anyone. However, it can be especially difficult if you've prided yourself on being a perfectionist or you're always on the go.

If you're the sort of person who gets things done and is always called on to complete a project on time, make the cookies for the bake sale or coach the Little League team, being unable to do your part because of your pain can be devastating.

When chronic pain hits, an overachiever often has to settle for being just like everyone else. This causes some people to fall victim to all-or-nothing thinking. If they can't head the committee, they don't even want to be involved. They completely dismiss themselves from their normal activities and become withdrawn and depressed.

Emotional cycle

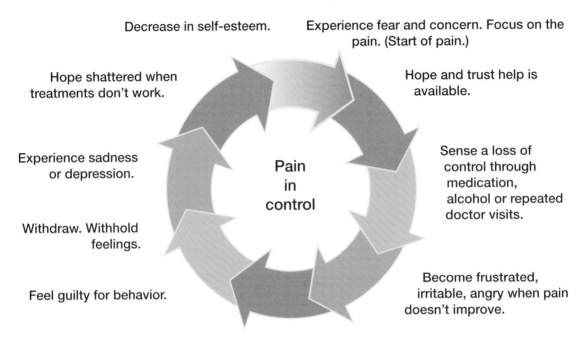

Uncontrolled chronic pain commonly causes this pattern of emotions, beginning at the top of the circle and moving clockwise.

your attempt to deal with your pain, because no one else seems to be able to.

Stage 3: Anger and frustration

You become dejected and depressed. This is the stage when you ask, "Why me?" and "What did I do to deserve this?" You know the pain isn't a punishment but you feel you've done something wrong, and now you're paying the price.

You may become more irritable with the people who are trying their best to help you. You may also find it easy to vent your frustration on others — your doctors, your insurance representative, and even your own family and friends.

But it's displaced anger; you're really not upset at them. Instead, what's upsetting you may be the long waits at your doctor's office, the bill at the end of each visit, your increased dependence on others and a sense of loss of control.

Stage 4: Guilt and withdrawal

Eventually, you start to feel guilty over the things you've said and done. Instead of communicating this guilt, you may withdraw from people so that you won't take your anger out on them.

You also feel guilty because you aren't able to do your full share anymore. Your spouse or children have taken over some of your regular duties, such as parenting responsibilities, cleaning the house or raking the yard. At work, you can't keep up your normal pace and your co-workers are having to lend you a hand.

All of this upsets and frustrates you. But you've had enough of venting your frustrations and getting upset with people you shouldn't, so you find yourself withholding your emotions and keeping them all bottled up inside.

Stage 5: Renewed hope, followed by depression

Gradually, or perhaps rather suddenly, you begin to feel better. You're optimistic that your condition is finally improving. Excitedly, you start getting back into your old routine. But after a time, the pain returns and you become deeply disappointed and lose all hope of recovery. You feel depressed and can hardly make it out of bed in the morning. Things that used to matter to you, such as your appearance or attending family or social activities, don't seem important anymore.

You may begin to feel as though you're no longer loved or needed, and your self-esteem hits an all-time low. You may even begin to wonder if you're deserving of love and attention.

As you draw deeper inside yourself, your pain becomes the focus of all of your attention. Your life completely revolves around how you're feeling. Fear, isolation and depression, coupled with days of nothing to do, may make the pain feel even worse. Eventually, it becomes bad enough that it forces you to search for other forms of treatment, possibly setting you up for a repeat of the emotional cycle.

Your family's responses

Your pain and how you react to it don't affect just you. They also affect

Family behavioral cycle

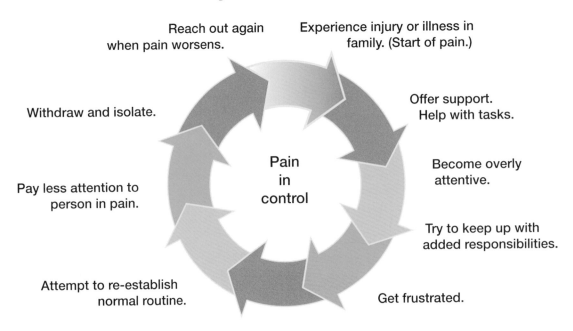

Reach out again when pain worsens.

Experience injury or illness in family. (Start of pain.)

Withdraw and isolate.

Offer support. Help with tasks.

Pain in control

Become overly attentive.

Pay less attention to person in pain.

Try to keep up with added responsibilities.

Attempt to re-establish normal routine.

Get frustrated.

Family emotional cycle

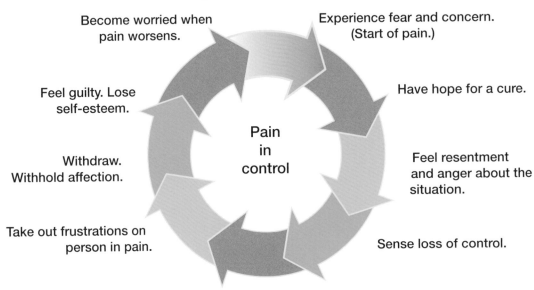

Become worried when pain worsens.

Experience fear and concern. (Start of pain.)

Feel guilty. Lose self-esteem.

Have hope for a cure.

Pain in control

Withdraw. Withhold affection.

Feel resentment and anger about the situation.

Take out frustrations on person in pain.

Sense loss of control.

Family members commonly experience patterns of behavior and emotion that are similar to those of the person in pain, beginning at the top of the circle and moving clockwise.

your family. So it's not surprising that your family's responses to your behaviors and emotions can take on parallel cycles of their own. Their reactions become similar to yours.

Family behaviors

When chronic pain first becomes a problem, family members generally show a great deal of support. They're often increasingly attentive to you, and they do more tasks around the house so that you can relax and "get better."

Family members also become vigilant in assessing your pain and keeping track of the activities that seem to make it better or worse. They observe and monitor you closely in an attempt to help lessen your pain and help your doctor make a diagnosis.

When your pain doesn't improve, your family's patience may start to wear thin. They begin to resent the extra burden they've been handed. And though most family members realize that it's not your fault, it becomes difficult to separate the person from the pain.

Family members may begin to withdraw and pay less attention to you. They become busy with their own lives.

Family emotions

Family members often go through the same emotions you do. Initially, they fear the cause of your pain. Later, when your treatment doesn't seem to be working and they're shouldering more responsibilities, they become angry and begin to ask, "Why me?" — or more appropriately, "Why us?"

Similar to you, family members often feel a loss of control over their daily lives. This frustration can lead them to withhold affection because they're angry at the situation facing them. They may unintentionally take this anger out on you.

They feel bad about being angry with you and, in turn, start to feel bad about themselves and how they're acting. "I'm not a good person" and "I should be able to handle this" are common thoughts. Their guilt often leads to increased attentiveness and care, beginning the emotional cycle again.

While you and your family share common feelings, you may find these feelings difficult to talk about. Family members fear it will sound as if they're blaming you. They also don't want to come across as being selfish and inconsiderate. The silence becomes frustrating.

Breaking the cycles

You may think that the cycles of chronic pain will never end, but you can break free of them. The downward spiral that often accompanies chronic pain occurs when all of your attention is focused on your pain.

By learning how to manage your pain, you're able to move your pain from the forefront — so that it no longer is the focus of your attention. As a result, you can concentrate on those things that give you pleasure and satisfaction. This renewed feeling will put you in control of your life instead of letting your pain control your life.

In upcoming chapters, we discuss a number of steps that you can take to get relief from your pain and break free from the pain cycles.

Chapter 5

The toll of chronic pain

The financial effects of persistent pain are evident in health care costs, demand for rehabilitation services and lost worker productivity. Unrelieved pain can result in longer hospital stays, increased rates of re-hospitalization, increased outpatient visits and a decreased ability to function fully, leading to lost income and insurance coverage.

According to an Institute of Medicine report *Relieving Pain in America: A Blueprint for Transforming Prevention, Care, Education, and Research*, pain is a significant public health problem that affects about 100 million American adults and costs society up to $635 billion annually.

For some families, medical bills, medications, lost days of work or an inability to work can greatly strain their finances. Some people reach a point where they need to see a financial consultant, move to a less expensive home, or cash in all of their savings to avoid bankruptcy.

But chronic pain is often more than just a financial burden. The emotional and physical toll the condition can cause, can be very costly as well. This chapter details some of the personal costs associated with chronic pain. It's not an upbeat discussion. But the good news is that the story doesn't end here.

This book is about improving your personal health and quality of life, despite your pain. The chapters that follow outline what you can do to help minimize these personal costs and, in some cases, avoid them.

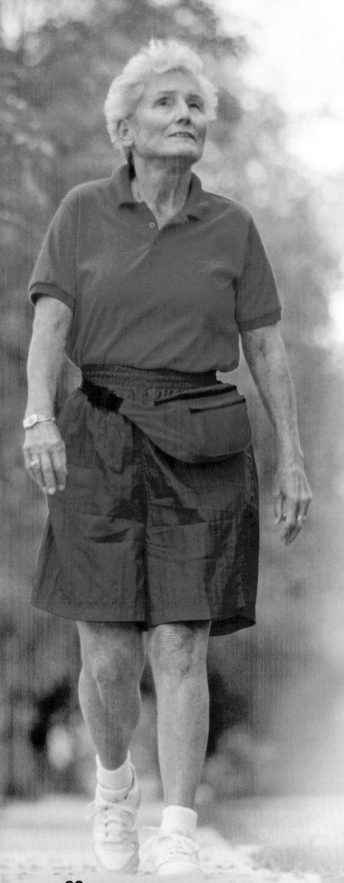

Physical deconditioning

You know that you need regular physical activity to stay healthy. But when you're in pain, you don't feel like being active. Like many people, you may have started an exercise routine, but you did too much the first day. The next day you felt so much worse that the thought of exercising again was more than you could handle. So, you didn't. The day after, it wasn't any easier to get up and get moving, and pretty soon you found yourself doing less and less.

Inactivity generally leads to increased body fat. In addition to weight gain, a higher proportion of body fat increases your risk of cardiovascular disease and diabetes. Inactivity can also weaken your bones and elevate your risk of osteoporosis. As your body becomes more deconditioned, you may feel as though you'll never be healthy again.

Regular physical activity is crucial to pain control. But it's important that you perform the right kinds of exercise and that you moderate your activity. For more on the role of exercise in managing chronic pain, see Chapter 12.

Loss of sleep

Chronic pain interferes with restful sleep. According to the National Sleep Foundation, approximately two-thirds of people with chronic pain report poor, unrefreshing sleep.

In addition to the direct effect of pain on sleep, other factors associated with chronic pain can indirectly influence how much and how well you rest:

Lack of physical activity. Inactivity makes it more difficult for you to relax and sleep well.

Excessive alcohol. Drinking too much alcohol reduces the amount of restful sleep you get by interfering with your brain's ability to produce adequate periods of deep sleep.

Medications. Some pain medications contain caffeine, which can stimulate your nervous system, so you don't feel tired.

When you don't get adequate sleep, you lack energy, you're more easily irritated, and you aren't able to cope as well with pain and stress. Regular or extended bouts of sleeplessness can also wear on your health in other ways.

For more information on the association between sleep and chronic pain, as well as tips to help you sleep better, see page 202.

Emotional upheaval

Pain can play havoc with your emotions. One minute you may feel fine, the next your world may feel as though it's been torn apart. For some people, a specific event — such as an accident or a fall — can change their life in an instant. For others, the development of chronic pain is a more gradual process. In either case, the pain has divided your life into two distinct parts — life as you knew it before the pain and life as you now know it with pain.

In your new life, you may feel powerless and trapped. Your emotions may range from fear and frustration to anger and apathy. Dealing with these emotions is often difficult. As you think back to life before your pain, you may become more angry or frustrated.

When you're in pain, your sense of security also may disappear. You may ask yourself: What if I lose my job? Will my family understand? What do my friends think of me? The more anxious you become, the more stressed you feel. For more on dealing with your emotions, see Chapter 15.

Depression

Chronic pain and depression often go hand in hand. Persistent pain, combined with emotional strain, may create a sinkhole that can be difficult to escape. The prevalence of depression in people with chronic pain is generally higher than it is in people with other medical disorders.

It's natural to experience some discouragement when your pain first develops and for short periods afterward. The pain itself also can cause symptoms such as slowed movements or loss of energy, often associated with depression. If your symptoms linger for several months or they become severe, it's important that you talk to a doctor. You may be experiencing depression.

A person with depression may have some, most or all of these symptoms:

- Lasting sadness
- Irritability and mood swings

- Loss of interest or pleasure in most activities
- Change in appetite and weight (gain or loss)
- Recurrent early awakening or other changes in sleep patterns
- Feelings of restlessness
- Feelings of hopelessness or helplessness
- Extreme fatigue, loss of energy or slowed movements
- Continual negative view of others and the world
- Feelings of worthlessness or inappropriate feelings of guilt
- Neglect of personal responsibilities and care
- Decreased concentration, attention and memory
- Decreased sex drive
- Increased focus on physical complaints
- Thoughts of death or suicide

The fundamental causes of depression aren't fully understood, but psychological and biological factors are both important. Genetic factors, imbalances in certain body or brain chemicals, or abnormal sleep behaviors also may give rise to depression. In addition, living with chronic pain and having to give up enjoyable and pleasurable activities can trigger depression.

Regardless of the cause, depression is a complex condition that can make your pain feel worse. People who are depressed often report stronger, longer lasting and more severe pain than do people who aren't depressed.

Treating depression can result in less pain or pain that's easier to manage. Treatment for depression is often very effective. However, many people don't receive treatment because they're unaware of their condition or they don't view depression as an illness. For more information on chronic pain and depression see page 225.

For more information on chronic pain and depression see page 225.

Difficulties at work and school

When your first started experiencing pain, your employer may have been sympathetic to you. Perhaps your boss made your workload lighter to accommodate you, or your co-workers

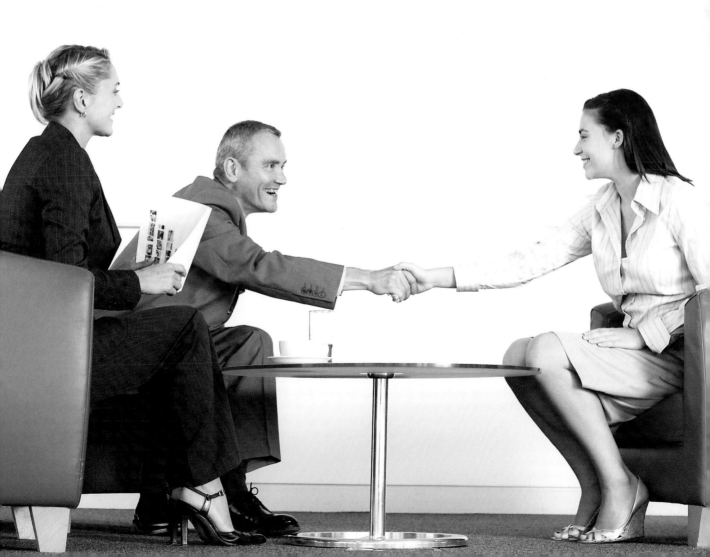

pitched in to help you out. But as your condition lingered, things changed. Your boss and co-workers were less willing to help you out.

Troubles with a boss or lack of understanding from co-workers can make work a stressful place. This only adds to the pain. If you're having trouble keeping up, you may also fear that you'll lose your job.

The result may be some difficult decisions. Steps that might help reduce your pain and your stress may involve requesting a shorter workday or changing jobs. That may not be possible or could involve some unacceptable compromises. For example, another, less stressful position may not offer a comparable salary or insurance benefits.

Chronic pain doesn't affect just adults. Kids experience chronic pain, too. For teens with persistent pain, one of the real costs of their condition is missed days of school. Some kids miss so much school that they eventually enroll in an alternative educational setting such as online learning or home school.

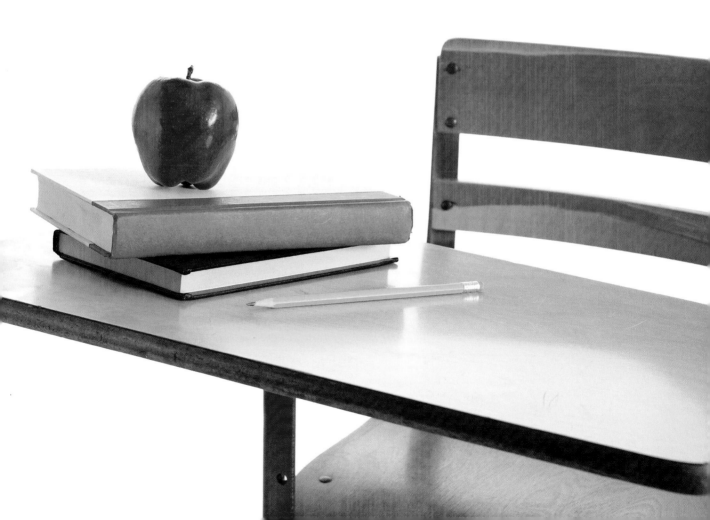

Damaged relationships

People who were once supportive and always offering to lend a hand may not be around as much. They've gone on with their lives and seem to have less time for you.

Family relationships also seem strained. Even though your family knows you're not to blame, they're frustrated for the way your pain has changed your life and theirs.

Communication may be difficult. You may find yourself taking out your emotions on those closest to you. Or, to the contrary, you withdraw and don't share your thoughts or feelings.

Your pain may also be straining your sexual relationship. Some people experience sexual difficulties due to their pain or stress, or as a side effect of medications they take to relieve pain or associated conditions. Others avoid intimacy and sexual intercourse because they no longer feel sexually attractive or they fear intercourse will increase their pain.

For more on managing personal relationships, see Chapter 17.

Substance misuse

It's not uncommon for people who are in pain to turn to drugs to help relieve the pain. Reliance on medications and substances such as alcohol or illicit drugs can be a troublesome side effect of chronic pain. Some signs of substance misuse include:

- A preoccupation with taking medications
- Taking more medication than prescribed
- Use of more than one doctor or pharmacy to get medication
- Hiding medications or being secretive about their use
- Using someone else's medication
- Frequent use of an emergency room to get medication
- Using alcohol or illicit drugs, including marijuana, to treat pain

Similar to prescription medications, misuse of alcohol or illicit drugs as a way to relieve pain and daily pressures can lead to chemical dependency. Plus, when you combine prescription medications with other drugs, including alcohol, you increase your risk of dangerous side effects.

For more on drug dependence and the misuse of medications, see Chapter 7.

Taking it one step at a time

Overcoming the costs of your pain may seem daunting. But remember that the problems that chronic pain can produce are often linked. Taking even a few small steps can bring noticeable results. For example, making an effort to reduce daily stress can have a positive effect on your physical health, sleep, work, personal relationships, finances and depression. As you begin to see improvements, the challenges ahead may seem less daunting.

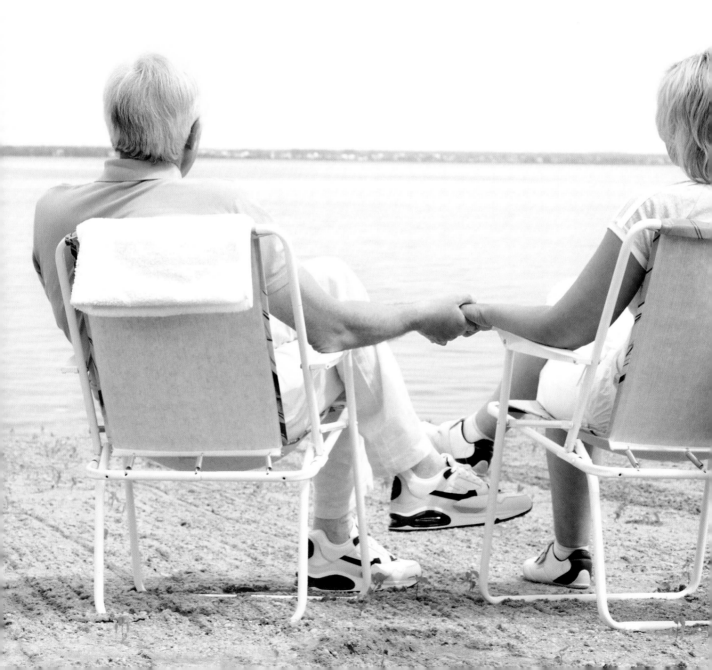

Chapter 6

Kids and chronic pain

Being a kid and living with chronic pain isn't that unusual. Like adults, children and adolescents experience everyday hurts that are unpleasant. But quite a few kids live with the kind of pain that's always sort of in the background or pain that comes and goes but never really goes away.

Pain may affect a specific part of the body, as joint pain, headaches or abdominal pain. It can also involve many regions of the body at once, as in generalized body pain.

For kids experiencing constant pain, the pain is more than simple bumps and bruises. And in many cases, these kids develop difficulties carrying on their regular activities and routines. Some kids also experience depression, medication side effects or anxiety. For

these young people, life just isn't the same anymore.

If you know or have a child that's dealing with chronic pain, this chapter is for you. You'll learn what types of chronic pain are most common in kids, the effects chronic pain can have on your child's life and your family life, how the pain can be managed, and what you can do to move on in spite of the pain.

Common types of pain

Chronic pain in children can range from something as familiar as a headache to the rarer facial pain. Surveys of thousands of different kids and research from chronic pain clinics suggest that the most common types of chronic pain in children and adolescents include headaches (also the most studied type), abdominal pain, and muscular and joint pain. Other common forms include generalized pain and complex regional pain syndrome.

Headaches

Based on surveys, about 1 out of every 4 kids experiences headache at least once a week. One type of headache is migraine, which can cause pain so sharp that all your child can think about is finding a dark, quiet place to lie down. It can also make him or her feel nauseated and want to throw up.

Another common type of headache is tension type. This kind of headache can make your child feel as if his or her head is wrapped in a tight band. When headache occurs more than 15 days a month for more than three months, it's called chronic daily headache.

Abdominal pain

Estimates vary widely, but up to 1 in 5 kids experiences persistent abdominal pain. A smaller percentage of kids experiences abdominal pain that's bad enough to keep them from doing regular activities, such as going to school or playing sports. In some kids, abdominal pain goes hand in hand with headache or back pain. Some kids lose their appetites and have difficulty eating, resulting in weight loss. While for others, abdominal pain may lead to weight gain.

Muscular and joint pain

Another common type of chronic pain affects your muscles and joints (musculoskeletal pain). Back pain is one example. Some studies indicate that about 1 in 5 kids experiences back pain at least once a month. Other studies have found that 1 out of every 5 kids has back pain every week.

Complex regional pain syndrome

Some kids experience a type of chronic pain, usually in a leg or an arm, called complex regional pain syndrome (CRPS). In addition to intense burning pain, the leg or arm may be sensitive to touch, feel cooler than other parts of the body and appear swollen. In many cases, the cause of the pain can't be explained. Generally, doctors think it may be a result of the body's nervous system being overly sensitive to stimuli. Similar to other chronic pain conditions, CRPS can be a challenge because there's no single test that can diagnose it, making it more difficult and time-consuming to evaluate and treat.

Generalized pain

This kind of chronic pain can affect children and adolescents, as well as adults. In addition to causing general achiness, this type of pain can make your child feel extremely tired, even after sleeping for a long period of time. Sleep itself is often restless and disrupted by movement of legs or arms and periodic waking.

Unknown pain

For some kids, the cause of their pain is never discovered. But this doesn't mean that the pain isn't real or that it doesn't require management. For these children and their families, the situation can be especially frustrating. They've often been through countless evaluations, seen a host of specialists and tried any number of treatments.

Disruptions to daily life

Kids respond to chronic pain in a variety of ways. For many of them, the pain is a mild nuisance and it doesn't prevent them from going to school and doing the things they enjoy.

For some kids, chronic pain brings with it a more pervasive set of problems. As with adults, kids can get stuck in a pain cycle that undermines their ability to move confidently through daily activities. Realizing there may be no quick fix for the pain can make both a child and a parent feel as if they've lost control, increasing frustration and sadness and decreasing the ability to focus on anything else while looking for a cure.

As a parent, your first instinct is to protect your child when he or she is hurting. But focusing solely on your child's pain while overlooking other aspects of life can have some serious unintended consequences. Take a look at the toll chronic pain can take on a child's life.

Loss of routine

If your child wakes up in pain, it's natural for you to tell your child to stay

When your child has POTS

Kids that come to Mayo Clinic's Pediatric Pain Rehabilitation Program have a variety of chronic pain disorders. Headache (30 percent) and abdominal pain (32 percent) are the most frequent pain disorders. But a significant percentage of kids (31 percent) also have a diagnosis of postural orthostatic-tachycardic syndrome (POTS).

What is it?

POTS is a condition that occurs when your autonomic nervous system doesn't work as it should. Your autonomic nerves control your involuntary body functions such as your blood pressure and heart rate. Nerve fibers in your autonomic nervous system normally direct how fast your heart needs to pump blood, where that blood needs to go and how it should flow. With POTS, these nerves may fire differently, so blood may pool in the legs more than normal upon standing. This produces a variety of signs and symptoms, one of which is postural orthostatic tachycardia — a heart rate that speeds up excessively when you go from a sitting to a standing position. This can make you feel faint and lightheaded.

Other common symptoms may include chest pain, shortness of breath, vision problems, fatigue, weakness, headache, nausea, bloating, sleep problems, sweating, and heat or cold intolerance.

POTS often begins in the early teen years and is typically triggered by a serious injury or illness, such as a viral infection. Symptoms of POTS can vary widely from one person to the next. For example, some teens experience mild symptoms most of the time. Others also experience "storms," periods where many symptoms converge and then lessen.

Getting to a diagnosis

If you're a parent of a child with POTS, you're probably all too familiar with emergency rooms, doctor's offices, tests and more tests. It's not easy dealing with the uncertainty that often precedes a diagnosis of POTS. Because the symptoms can indicate any number of medical conditions, people with POTS may go through many evaluations and see many health care providers before arriving at a diagnosis.

Once POTS is suspected, however, the diagnosis can be made using a tilt table test. During the test, you lie on an examination table that's tilted into different positions. Changes in your heart rate and blood pressure are recorded with changes in position.

Managing symptoms

The good news is most teens grow out of POTS by the time they reach early adulthood. In the meantime, the condition can be managed with diet, exercise and medications. Increasing fluid and salt intake on a daily basis enhances blood flow, while regular aerobic exercise increases energy and helps retrain the autonomic nervous system to regulate blood flow correctly. Medications, such as beta blockers, may be prescribed to improve heart rate, chest pain and irregular heartbeats. Some kids also benefit from talking to a counselor or other support person, to help them deal with anxiety, sadness or just the stress of coping with a chronic condition.

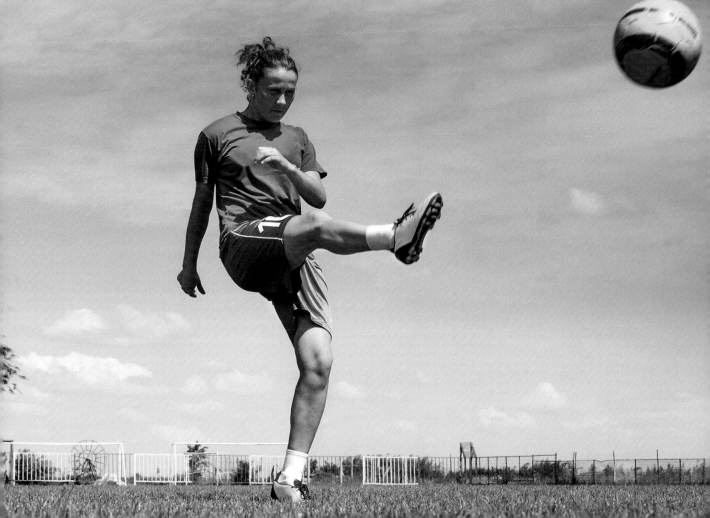

at home until he or she feels better. But with chronic pain, this can happen so often that your child is missing several days of school a month or even a week. Pain becomes the sole deciding factor for whether your child gets up and goes to school or goes to play practice or a soccer game. An erratic schedule can also lead to irregular sleep patterns, which can lead to loss of energy and irritability.

Social and developmental losses

Not only does missing school represent an academic loss, it results in missed opportunities for your child to socialize and hang out with his or her friends. And the more your child is isolated, the less likely he or she will be to try to catch up with friendships. School is also an environment that promotes achievement of developmental milestones, such as learning to manage time and developing personal responsibility.

Emotional stress and upheaval

Realizing how much the pain is robbing your child and your family life can make everyone involved feel stressed. Grieving the loss of a previous way of life and wondering what will come next adds to the family's anxiety and can lead to anger and resentment. Some children, and even parents, start to feel hopeless and depressed, which can lead to further withdrawal and isolation.

Physical deconditioning

It's easy to let your child withdraw from physical activities for fear of increasing pain symptoms. But this can result in rest that never ends. The less active your child becomes, the less equipped he or she is to handle even small amounts of activity. Called deconditioning, this lack of activity can lead to a downward spiral of fatigue, depression, stress and muscle tension. This, in turn, produces increased pain, starting the cycle all over again.

Managing chronic pain

Many families who have kids with chronic pain have gone through extensive searches for the cause of their child's pain. They may have seen

What are pain behaviors?

Pain behaviors are the things your child might say or do that signal he or she is in pain. Examples might include wincing, groaning or frequently talking about pain. More subtle pain behaviors might include avoiding others, being irritable with family and friends, and avoiding activities.

Pain behaviors are a natural response to acute pain, but with chronic pain they can become a habit. Your child may exhibit pain behaviors to get you to share in his or her discomfort or to draw attention and support from others.

The problem is pain behaviors become a constant reminder of pain, and they consume a great deal of energy. To increase your child's confidence and ability to cope with chronic pain, try to discourage pain behaviors.

When your child exhibits pain behaviors, it's easy for your reactions to fall into one of two categories:

- **Lenient.** You attempt to ease the pain or pain behavior by assuming your child's responsibilities or eliminating his or her chores, for example.
- **Critical.** You blame your child for his or her behavior with a response such as "Oh, no! Not this again."

To move the focus away from the pain, try taking a balanced approach and remaining neutral toward pain behaviors. This doesn't mean you're unsympathetic. It just means you don't respond to the behavior.

A neutral approach allows your child to develop his or her own course of action in response to chronic pain. Strategies your child can use to cope more effectively with chronic pain include relaxation techniques, a cool compress, thinking about pain differently or engaging in a fun activity. Some kids may not need help once they've learned these coping techniques, but others may find it helpful if a parent reminds them to use pain management strategies.

multiple doctors, therapists and other specialists and endured a range of tests and evaluations. As a parent of a child with chronic pain, you may have had experiences with medical professionals who seemed as if they didn't listen to your concerns, or who may have implied that chronic pain is not a real health issue.

Chronic pain is real. What's important to realize is that even if a cause or a cure is never found, the pain can be managed in such a way that you and your child and your family can still have a life despite the pain.

Ironically, as you start doing the things you have to and want to do, the pain may lessen. It's best not to pay too much attention to your daily pain level. Chances of improvement seem to be best when your pain isn't the focus of your attention.

Parts 2 and 3 of this book are all about treating and managing chronic pain. Much of the information is applicable to kids and teens, as well as adults. Browsing through the chapters will give you useful coping tools, but there are some issues specific to kids with chronic pain, which you can read about here.

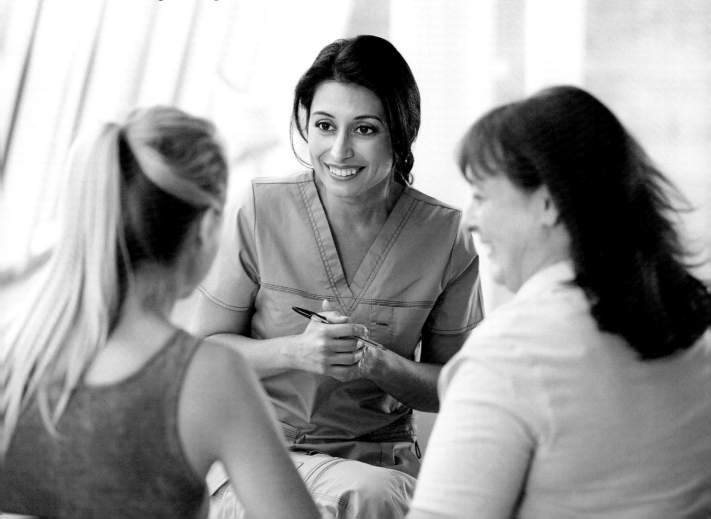

Find a doctor you trust

Whether you're pursuing a diagnosis for your child's pain or you've already arrived at one — even if the cause is unexplained — it's vital that you and your child have a relationship with a health professional you can trust. Preferably, this is a doctor experienced in helping kids with chronic pain. But at a minimum it should be a person who:

- Knows your child's history
- Is willing to help you find ways to improve your child's quality of life, including appropriate referrals to other specialists, such as a physical or occupational therapists
- Can help your family develop a chronic pain management plan
- Is attentive to your child's whole health, including evaluating and treating conditions unrelated to chronic pain but that might otherwise be overlooked

Having a doctor who you feel is an ally and a partner in overseeing your child's health can help ease some of the stress of worrying about your child's condition. A caring and thoughtful health professional can also help allay fears that you're missing something important or that you're not doing enough.

Approach medications with caution

When used appropriately, medications are useful. For some people and in certain situations, they can help reduce pain with limited side effects. Pain relievers may be used to control pain that's more intense than usual. In addition, medications often can effectively treat other conditions that may accompany chronic pain, such as depression or anxiety.

In general, though, medications can't cure chronic pain and they shouldn't be viewed as the answer to pain. Among other things, long-term use of medications can create its own set of problems, including increased pain. Overuse of pain relievers to treat headaches, for example, can lead to further headaches resulting from medication overuse.

With certain medications, there's also the risk of abuse. Misuse of medications, a serious and growing problem, is discussed beginning on page 110.

For most kids, what they do each day — exercising, eating well, using relaxation and mind and body therapies, following a daily routine, and going to school — does more to help beat chronic pain than does a daily dose of medication.

7 steps to getting back into life

You can help your child cope with chronic pain by encouraging him or her to engage in strategies that will put pain in proper focus and free up mental and physical energy for other more enjoyable aspects of life. Studies show that replacing dysfunctional behaviors, such as pain behaviors (see page 73), with more adaptive ones, such as positive thinking, can result in significantly less pain, a better quality of life and better general health.

When parents approach a child's chronic pain with the goal of keeping the child's life as normal and productive as possible, everyone — child, parents and the entire family — benefits. Children, and their parents, report decreased pain and less interference with their daily activities.

Following are key concepts used in Mayo Clinic's Pediatric Pain Rehabilitation Program. They're designed to promote active engagement in life and successful self-management of pain.

The majority of adolescents who've gone through the program indicated that they "agree" or "strongly agree" that the program was beneficial in helping them learn to live well in spite of pain. But you don't have to go through the program to benefit from the strategies it employs.

Read through the steps that follow and think about what might help you and your child better cope with chronic pain.

1. Send your child to school

Kids thrive on consistency and school is an important constant in almost every child's life. In addition to the academic gains, going to school every day provides your child with a number of benefits. For one, it provides structure to your child's day. Irregular sleep, unpredictable meal schedules and erratic activity levels can wear your child down and drain his or her energy, both of which can make pain worse. Attending school can help your child:

- Get up at the same time every morning
- Eat meals at the same time each day
- Reconnect with friends
- Avoid boredom
- Focus on something other than pain

If your child has been absent from school for a long time, it may be best for your child to return gradually — perhaps attending school for an hour or two a day the first week, then gradually increasing to half days and whole days.

Work with school staff to develop a plan for your child to manage his or her pain at school that follows the same guidelines as the plan you use at home. For example, at peak pain periods, your child might lie down for a few moments in the nurse's office or retreat to a quiet place in the school to practice relaxation strategies. In general, you want to avoid:

- **Having school staff send your child home due to pain.** Ask them to treat your child as much like any other child as possible.
- **Requesting a reduced workload.** If your child has missed a significant amount of school due to chronic pain, he or she should work with teachers to develop a reasonable plan for making up missed schoolwork.
- **Allowing your child to miss school because of pain, even if it's a little worse than usual.** In rare cases, if pain forces your child to miss school

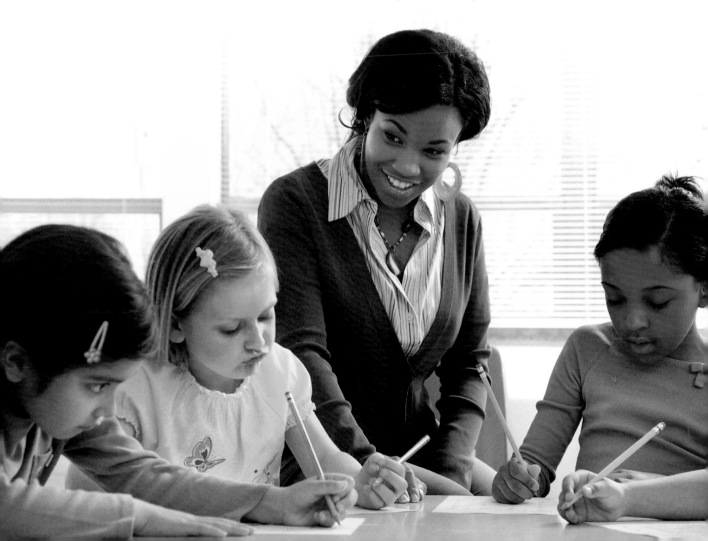

if he or she can't do chores or is unable to fulfill other responsibilities, don't allow privileges, such as watching television, playing games or doing other activities.

2. Encourage exercise

People often think that getting up and moving around or exercising can make pain worse. In reality, exercise can help your child feel better. It can take the edge off of the pain and ease feelings of stress, sadness and frustration.

Exercise is important because it:

- Causes the body to release chemicals that help block pain impulses from reaching the brain (endorphins)
- Strengthens muscles and increases flexibility
- Lowers stress hormones

Encourage your child to exercise or better yet, exercise with him or her. Try walking, swimming or biking — whatever you enjoy doing together. Start out slow and gradually increase the time as your child develops more stamina.

Why go through all the effort?

Sometimes you or your child may wonder why go through all the effort of exercising, eating and sleeping well, practicing relaxation, and going to school when the pain is still there?

But what you do matters. Your body sends pain signals through a system of nerves in your brain and spinal cord. To stop these signals from reaching their destination, your body releases its own painkilling chemicals, called endorphins, to help block pain signals.

Positive thoughts and feelings, physical activity, relaxation, and healthy relationships all help boost your body's ability to release the endorphins needed to block pain signals and retrain your body's nerve pathways to respond in ways that lessen pain. They also influence how you cope with painful or stressful situations.

At first, your child may experience an increase in pain. Don't let that stop him or her from exercising.

3. Practice mind and body therapies

Mind and body medicine uses the power of the mind to improve health. Mind and body therapies are more than simple distractions. They help relieve pain by eliminating tension and preventing muscle spasms. They also alter the body's chemistry by decreasing its production of stress hormones and increasing its release of pain-fighting chemicals such as endorphins and enkephalins (see Chapters 10 and 16).

4. Help your child sleep and eat well

Getting a good night's sleep can help your child feel refreshed and ready to

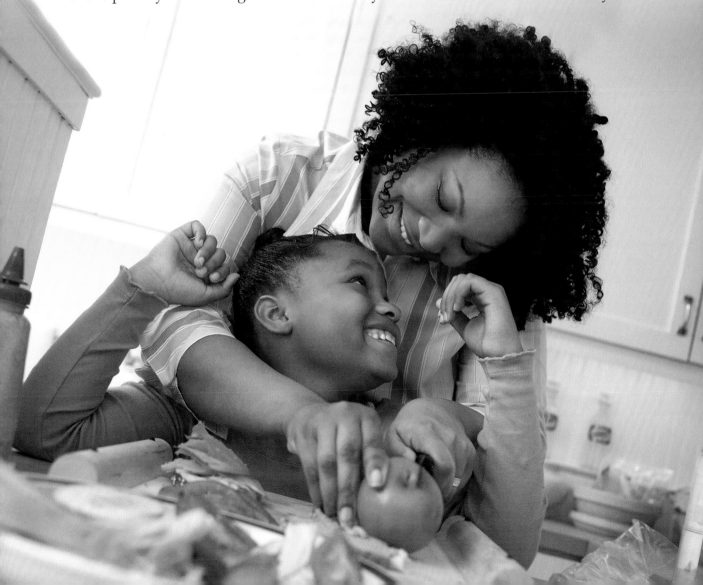

face the day. Most teens, for example, need 8½ to 9½ hours of sleep a night to feel rested. Younger children typically need slightly more sleep.

Trying to fall asleep when you're in pain can be frustrating, though. To maximize your child's chances of getting a good night's rest, consider these tips:

- Maintain a consistent bedtime and waking time. Sleeping in an extra hour on the weekends is OK, but too much more than that can interfere with sleep cycles.
- Keep the bedroom cool, dark and quiet at nighttime.
- Have your child stay away from pop, sugar and big meals before bedtime. Skip caffeine after 4 p.m.
- Avoid keeping a TV, computer, cellphone or other electronic devices in the bedroom, which can distract from sleep.
- Help your child clear his or her mind by writing down impending to-do items or creating a list of action items for the next day.

Eating a balanced diet is also important because it can give your child more energy and help him or her maintain a healthy weight. Encourage your son or daughter to eat more fruit, vegetables and whole grains. Go easy on soda and processed foods such as chips and cookies. Serve moderate portions.

5. Respond consistently

Two parents in the same house can have very different styles and strategies for dealing with a child who has

Plan ahead for difficult days

Even after your child has learned to manage pain, he or she will still have difficult days on occasion. Together, make a plan for these times. Decide what strategies to employ when the pain gets bad and where your child can go to relax, including at school. The goal is to minimize disruptiveness and return to everyday activities as quickly as possible. See Chapter 18 for tips on setting up a pain management plan for difficult days.

When to consider a pain rehab program

If you've tried everything, including the suggestions in this chapter, and nothing is really working, you might consider enrolling in a pediatric pain rehabilitation program. These programs incorporate multiple disciplines, including pain specialists, physical and occupational therapists, and psychologists.

Pain rehabilitation programs are proven ways of improving quality of life, physical conditioning and depression. They can also help your child discontinue medications and return to school and social and recreational activities. Generally, parents are involved in a portion of the program, as well.

If you're wondering whether a pain rehab program is right for your child, ask yourself these questions:
- Is my child's life focused on pain and what he or she is not able to do, rather than what he or she is able to do in spite of the pain?
- Is my child missing school and social events due to pain?
- Are my child's doctors telling me there is nothing further they can do to relieve the pain? Do they tell me that we need to learn to get on with life?
- Am I truly concerned about the long-term effects of my child taking pain medications?
- Is my family's well-being affected because of my child's chronic pain?
- Is my child's recovery from injury or illness taking much longer than his or her doctors or I expected?
- Is my child not able to commit to sports or social events because his or her pain may be higher that day?

If you answered yes to one or more of these questions, then a pediatric pain rehab program may be appropriate.

chronic pain. Because consistency is important, talk with your partner about how you'll handle your child's pain behaviors. If you find it difficult to agree, talk to a supportive third party, such as your child's doctor or a family therapist.

In addition to responding consistently, it's important for parents to lean on and support each other during difficult times. Turn toward your marriage even as you work to increase your child's confidence and independence in managing chronic pain.

6. Help siblings cope

When a child with pain becomes the focus of all the parents' attention, brothers and sisters may feel isolated, angry or jealous. They may also feel guilty for having these feelings.

As regularly as possible, try to spend one-on-one time with all of your children and be open to talking to them about their brother's or sister's chronic pain. Encourage your other children to express how it affects them. Talk about how your other children can help your child with pain feel more upbeat and positive and how they can provide distractions when appropriate.

7. Have fun

Focusing on your child's pain can make you forget about activities and outings you used to enjoy, both with your child and as a family. Regularly take time to do something fun, whether it's taking a full-blown vacation or just pausing to be silly and laugh.

Remind yourself that your child isn't defined by chronic pain. Sit back and take stock of his or her evolving identity: What's unique about your child's personality? What are the things that make her tick? What makes him laugh? What are your child's strengths? Capitalize on those.

Enjoy your time together.

Part 2

Treating chronic pain

Chapter 7

Medication

Advances in medicine and technology have created a wide range of options for treating chronic pain. The most common form of treatment, however, remains medication.

When used appropriately, medications can help reduce pain, and some people experience only limited, if any, side effects from medication use. Medications can also help control a temporary flare in your pain. In addition, medications may be prescribed to help treat other conditions that can accompany chronic pain, such as depression, anxiety and sleep problems.

This chapter examines the role of medications in treating chronic pain. It also offers suggestions on how to get the most from your medications. In the pages that follow, you'll find information about specific types of drugs to treat pain, including:

- Simple pain relievers
- Opioids (narcotics)
- Topical medications
- Other pain medications
- Medications for emotional symptoms
- Medications for other physical conditions

Understanding pain medications

The role of medications in treating chronic pain is complex and sometimes controversial. There are many kinds of medications, and doctors have varying opinions about them and how they should be used.

In part, the controversy results from the very nature of chronic pain. Treating persistent pain can be more difficult than treating acute pain, which is often short term with a clear cause.

To prescribe medications that effectively help with chronic pain, your doctor has to consider and balance a number of factors. Knowing what these factors are may help you better understand your treatment plan.

Rehabilitation
Treatment of chronic pain shouldn't simply aim at controlling symptoms. The larger goal is to help you lead a full and active life.

Efficacy
This term refers to the power of a medication to produce desired results — in this case, a reduction in the level of pain. Higher doses of a medication may not increase its efficacy. And a higher dose, or the use of an additional medication, may increase the risk of side effects.

Safety
Pain medications can cause a variety of potentially serious side effects. The higher the dose or the longer you take the medication, generally the greater the risk of side effects. With some medications, you may develop a tolerance to the drug the longer you take it. Some serious side effects that may occur with use of pain medications include bleeding ulcers, liver damage and slowed breathing (decreased respirations).

Interactions
Your doctor will try to avoid drug combinations that cause unsafe interactions — unwanted effects that can occur when some drugs are taken together. Equally important is preventing drug-disease interactions — prescribing a drug for chronic pain that may worsen another condition, such as diabetes. Finally, interactions with over-the-counter medications, alcohol and certain foods also may cause problems.

Allergies
An allergy to one pain medication may eliminate an entire class of drugs that could be used in your treatment.

Life situation
To understand this factor, compare two people. One is an older adult with high levels of pain due to end-stage cancer. Another is a middle-aged person with chronic back pain who still maintains a full work schedule and has a busy family life. The person with cancer

may have a treatment plan that calls for higher doses of medication to deliver immediate pain relief. The second person may need to balance medication dosage and pain relief with safety and the ability to function in daily life.

Placebo effects
If you try a new pain medication, you might feel better at first, even though the new medication has no specific advantage over a previously used medication. This is the placebo effect, and it can complicate treatment of chronic pain.

Practical issues
You and your doctor need to consider the cost of your medication and the challenges of sticking to a medication schedule. Some pain medications are short acting and must be taken several times a day. Other medications have longer lasting effects and can be taken less often.

In light of these factors, your doctor likely will want to tailor your medication to your specific needs and circumstances, applying the concept of hierarchical treatment. This means that your treatment may take place in stages. You may begin with fewer medications in lower doses. You and your doctor will judge how well this approach works

before trying stronger medications, adding to the number of medications or increasing the doses, at the risk of more side effects.

Remember that medication is usually just one option in a full treatment plan. Your plan may also include physical therapy, counseling and lifestyle changes. Some people find these other therapies help reduce or eliminate their need for pain medication.

If you take pain medication, you may not need it long term. Ask your doctor how long you may be on the medication and what the alternatives are if it's not helpful. If, after a designated period of time, you find that it doesn't seem to be providing much benefit, you might discuss with your doctor if it's worth continuing to take it.

Medication use

To get the most from your medications, it's important to be actively involved in your care. The following steps can increase the safety and efficacy of your medications.

Share information
Your doctor needs to know exactly which medications you take. Keep an

up-to-date list of all of your medications. It might be best to keep your medications in their original containers and bring them along when you see your doctor. Include both prescription and nonprescription medications, as well as dietary supplements and herbs.

It's also important that you use only one pharmacy to fill your prescription medications. By knowing all of the medications you take, your pharmacist can watch out for potentially dangerous drug interactions.

With all medications you take — both prescription and over-the-counter — know these details:

- **Name of medication.** To avoid confusion, remember that medications have both generic and brand names.
- **Dosage.** Dosage refers to the strength of medication you take at one time and how often you take the medication.
- **Purpose.** Why did you begin taking the medication? For example, was it prescribed to treat your pain or to treat a condition associated with your pain, such as insomnia or depression?
- **How you take the medication.** Do you take the medication with or without food? Do you take it just

before going to bed or earlier in the day?
- **Results.** Do you feel or notice any unexpected side effects from the medication? How well do you think the drug is working? Keep in mind that some medications take time to work. It may take six months to find out if the drug is beneficial. If it's not, talk to your doctor about discontinuing its use.
- **Other health conditions.** If you're allergic to certain medications or think you might be pregnant, be sure to tell your doctor. Also mention any other illnesses or conditions you have.

Be informed
Keep and read all the printed materials that come with your medications. These materials offer general information that may answer some of your questions. Make sure you know exactly why you're taking the medication and what results you can expect.

Stick to your plan
Take your medication exactly as prescribed by your doctor. If you stop taking a drug before your prescription ends, you could undermine the results of your treatment. The same thing can happen if you cut down on a medication without consulting your doctor

or if you take more of a drug than prescribed.

Medication that worked well for you several months or years ago could have different effects on you today. Sometimes doses need to be changed or the whole treatment plan needs to be adjusted. Watch out for changes in your health and report those changes to your doctor.

Simple pain relievers

Simple pain relievers, also called analgesics, are medications designed to reduce or relieve pain. These drugs are often the first step in controlling pain.

They work in various ways, by interfering with the processes in which pain messages are developed, transmitted or interpreted. Simple analgesics are not the same as opioid medications — commonly referred to as narcotics — which are described later in this chapter.

Acetaminophen

Acetaminophen includes the brand-name drug Tylenol. It's most effective for mild to moderate pain that isn't accompanied by inflammation.

When taken occasionally and as recommended, acetaminophen is safe. The drug is generally considered less problematic than other simple pain relievers because it doesn't cause side effects such as stomach pain and bleeding. However, if you frequently take more

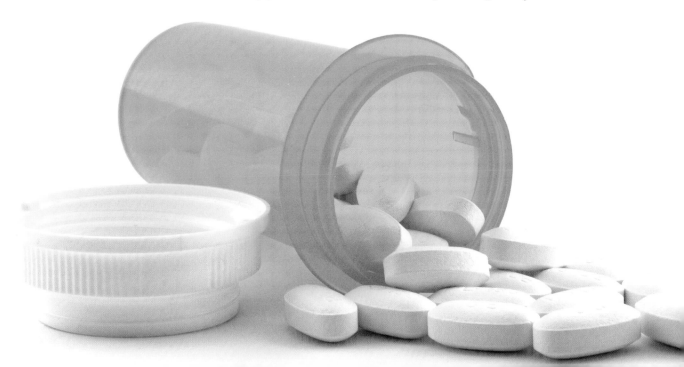

acetaminophen than recommended on the product label, you risk liver or kidney damage. Taking acetaminophen with alcohol also increases that risk and can lead to sudden and severe problems such as liver failure. In addition, unlike other pain relievers, acetaminophen does little to reduce inflammation.

Acetaminophen is sometimes combined with an opioid to provide stronger pain relief. These drugs are available only by prescription. Whenever you use a combination of medications, ask your doctor or pharmacist about the use and side effects of each drug.

Nonsteroidal anti-inflammatory drugs

Nonsteroidal anti-inflammatory drugs (NSAIDs) are most effective for mild to moderate pain that's accompanied by swelling and inflammation. They relieve pain by inhibiting an enzyme in your body called cyclooxygenase. This enzyme makes hormone-like substances called prostaglandins, which are involved in the development of pain and inflammation. NSAIDs are especially helpful for arthritis and pain resulting from muscle sprains, strains, back and neck injuries, or cramps.

There are several brands of NSAIDs sold by prescription. Nonprescription NSAIDs sold over-the-counter include ibuprofen (Advil, Motrin IB, others) and naproxen sodium (Aleve). Aspirin is sometimes referred to as an NSAID. However, aspirin is different from traditional NSAIDs. It works on slightly different molecular pathways and its side effects can be more severe.

When taken as directed, NSAIDs are generally safe. But if you take more than the recommended dosage — and sometimes even the recommended dosage — NSAIDs may cause nausea, stomach pain, stomach bleeding or ulcers. Large doses of NSAIDs can also lead to kidney problems, fluid retention and high blood pressure. Risk of these conditions increases with age. If you regularly take NSAIDs, talk to your doctor so that he or she can monitor you for side effects.

NSAIDs also have a so-called ceiling effect — a limit as to how much pain they can control. This means that beyond a certain dosage, they don't provide additional benefit. If you have moderate to severe pain, exceeding the dosage recommendations may not help to relieve your pain and may increase your risk of side effects.

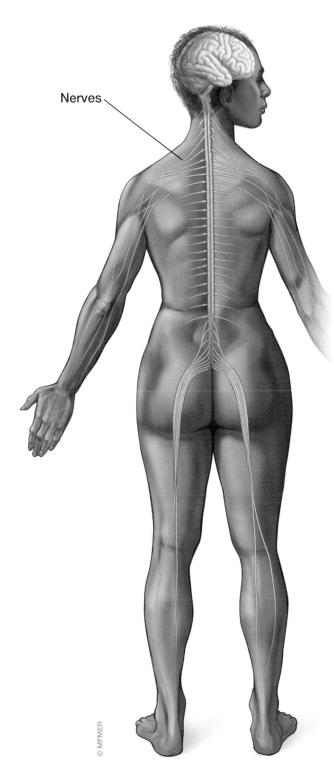

Nerves

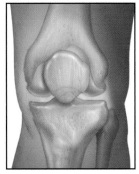

Normal knee

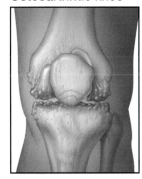

Osteoarthritic knee

NSAIDs

NSAIDs work in two ways. They reduce inflammation. They also alter the way in which the central nervous system — spinal cord and brain — interpret pain signals coming from the nerves so that the intensity of the pain signal is reduced or eliminated. NSAIDs are often used to reduce pain associated with inflammatory conditions, such as arthritis and muscle sprains.

COX-2 inhibitors

This class of medications is similar to NSAIDs, but the drugs work in a different manner. COX-2 inhibitors were developed with the aim of reducing some of the well-recognized side effects of traditional NSAIDs. Only one COX-2 inhibitor remains on the market, the drug celecoxib (Celebrex).

Like traditional NSAIDs, COX-2 inhibitors block production of the enzyme cyclooxygenase (COX). But unlike traditional NSAIDs, they affect only one form of the enzyme.

Cyclooxygenase comes in two forms — COX-1 and COX-2. Part of the role of COX-1 is to protect your stomach lining. Because NSAIDs suppress the function of COX-1, side effects such as stomach pain and bleeding problems can result. COX-2 inhibitors affect only COX-2, the form of the enzyme involved in the development of inflammation. Therefore, they cause fewer digestive problems, unless the medication is taken at higher dosages. Then the side effects are similar.

However, COX-2 inhibitors can still produce side effects, including symptoms of respiratory infection, headache and dizziness. And although the risk of stomach bleeding is generally lower if you take a COX-2 inhibitor instead of an NSAID, bleeding can still occur. In addition, these drugs can lead to kidney problems, fluid retention and high blood pressure. Older adults may be at higher risk of all of these side effects.

With both COX-2 inhibitors and traditional NSAIDs, the goal is to take the lowest effective dose for the shortest duration possible.

Opioids (narcotics)

Opioids, commonly called narcotics, are prescription medications that are regulated as controlled substances by the Drug Enforcement Administration. A doctor must have a special license in order to prescribe these medications.

Opioids are often used to relieve pain from cancer, terminal illness, severe injury or surgery. Pain control after surgery is especially important because the sooner you're active, the lower your risk of complications that can follow surgery, such as pneumonia or blood clots caused by inactivity.

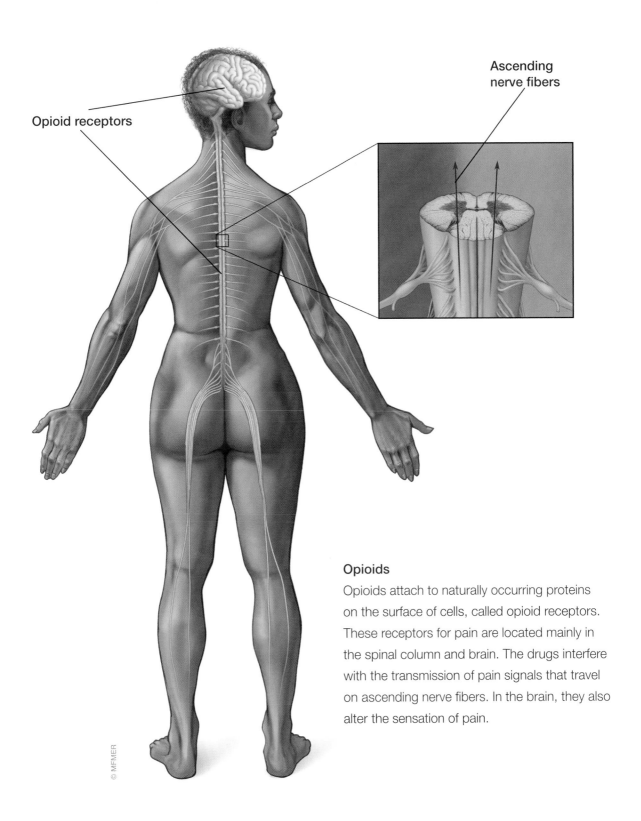

Opioid receptors

Ascending
nerve fibers

Opioids

Opioids attach to naturally occurring proteins
on the surface of cells, called opioid receptors.
These receptors for pain are located mainly in
the spinal column and brain. The drugs interfere
with the transmission of pain signals that travel
on ascending nerve fibers. In the brain, they also
alter the sensation of pain.

© MFMER

Opioids come in several forms. Some are natural compounds derived from the opium poppy plant. These compounds are called opiates. There are also synthetic opioids that work in similar ways. The term *opioids* refers to both natural and synthetic forms of the drug.

Most opioids are agonists, a drug that binds to a receptor of a cell and triggers a response by the cell. An agonist produces an action, whereas an antagonist acts against, or blocks, an action. Some opioid pain relievers are mixed agonists and antagonists — they work in two ways to relieve pain. Examples of mixed opioids include the drugs buprenorphine (Buprenex, Butrans), butorphanol (Stadol), levorphanol, nalbuphine and pentazocine (Talwin).

Opioid agonists, meanwhile, include:

- Codeine
- Fentanyl (Duragesic)
- Hydrocodone plus acetaminophen (Lortab, generic Vicodin)
- Hydromorphone (Dilaudid, Exalgo)
- Meperidine (Demerol)
- Methadone (Dolophine)
- Morphine (Avinza, MS Contin)
- Oxycodone (OxyContin, Roxicodone)
- Oxymorphone (Opana)

Side effects of opioids — particularly when the medications are taken at higher doses — include mild dizziness, drowsiness, sedation and unclear thinking. These effects can make it unsafe for you to drive, operate machinery or make important decisions.

Sometimes you can do things to manage the dizziness. For example, you might feel better after lying down for a while. If you experience severe dizziness or drowsiness, seek emergency care. Also go to the emergency room if you experience extreme nervousness or severe weakness, you have cold and clammy skin, or you have trouble breathing.

Other side effects of the medications include fatigue, constipation, nausea and vomiting. Ask your doctor or pharmacist about ways to manage these. In addition, opioids can lead to physical dependence or addiction.

Concerns about opioid use

With acute pain, the goal is to treat and relieve the pain as quickly as possible, usually with medication. Unrelieved pain has many negative effects, such as delayed recovery from surgery and decreased immunity to disease.

Understanding the risk of addiction

The issue of addiction is important, especially if you're taking an opioid medication. Many discussions about the effects of opioids get confused because people use three terms synonymously: tolerance, physical dependence and addiction. These words actually refer to three different conditions.

- **Tolerance.** Tolerance occurs when the initial dose of a narcotic loses its effectiveness over time. Some people refer to this as becoming "immune" to the drug. To get the same pain-relieving effect, you need to take higher doses of the medication. Unfortunately, in many cases, increasing the dose of the drug results in increased or unacceptable side effects.
- **Physical dependence.** This refers to the symptoms that result when your body becomes accustomed to a drug. When the drug is withdrawn, you may experience anxiety, tremors and other physical withdrawal symptoms. This happens in all people taking opioids if the medication is taken long enough.
- **Addiction.** Addiction is the term used to identify the irresistible craving for, loss of control over the use of, compulsive use of and continued use of a drug, despite repeated, harmful consequences. Drugs capable of producing addiction do so by interacting with the biochemistry of the brain in such a way that the drug seems essential — you feel the "need" for it just as you do food and water.

With time, people who take a narcotic are likely to develop tolerance and even physical dependence. However, this doesn't mean that they are, or will become, addicted to the drug. Most people treated with narcotics never experience addiction. Addiction results from many factors — genetic, psychological and environmental — and it often takes years to develop. Use of the drug is only one factor.

Sometimes, people with chronic pain act in ways that are mistakenly called addictive. These people may focus on maintaining their supply of opioids or closely watch the clock to make sure they take their next dose of medication. Often these are not addictive behaviors but pseudo-addiction — behaviors that stop once people get satisfactory pain relief.

For people with chronic pain, the goals of treatment are more complex. Pain relief is important, but so is the ability to function at work and to be able to enjoy social and leisure activities.

Sometimes, the goal of pain relief comes into conflict with the goal of improved physical functioning — especially when it comes to the use of opioids. Opioids are powerful pain relievers. When taken in small amounts and for short periods, they generally cause only minor side effects. But when opioids are taken in higher doses for several weeks or months, the side effects can impair your ability to function.

Opioids can also have an effect described as rebound pain. For instance, the effects of some opioids last only a few hours. Pain can recur as these short-acting medications wear off or when they're withdrawn from your treatment plan.

Opioids can also produce changes in your central nervous system that may heighten your perception of pain and make you feel more uncomfortable. This condition is called hyperalgesia.

In summary, opioids have many effects, some of them good and others not so good. For this reason — in addition to the fact that opioids aren't effective for all types of pain — some doctors prefer not to use opioids when treating chronic pain. These doctors may also be uneasy about possible long-term side effects of opioid use, which can interfere with rehabilitation and lead to more doctor visits and hospital stays. Doctors also cite the risk of physical dependence and addiction to the drugs. For more on misuse of prescription medications, especially opioids, see page 110.

Other doctors, meanwhile, take the position that withholding opioids may lead to unnecessary pain and suffering, that the side effects of opioids can be managed, and that the risk of addiction is overexaggerated. Doctors who hold this point of view on opioids believe that legal and medically supervised use of the medications has little in common with illegal use of such drugs.

If you take opioids

While there's debate about the use of opioids, these medications can be a key part of your treatment plan if your doctor feels that they can reduce your pain without causing severe side effects. Before prescribing an opioid, your doctor likely will get a detailed medical history and have you undergo a thorough physical examination. The results of the medical history and physical exam can help determine whether opioids are right for you.

If you're prescribed or you take a narcotic medication, consider your full range of options. Ask about the possibility of combining an opioid with a simple analgesic for maximum pain relief. Compare the benefits of short-acting and sustained-release medications. Discuss whether you should take the medications on a regular schedule or simply on an as-needed basis. You may also want to get a second opinion.

Finally, compare your mental and physical functioning and your activity levels with how you were getting along before you started the medication. If you haven't seen a marked improvement, it may not be worth continuing use of the drug.

Tramadol

Tramadol (Ultram) is a prescription pain medication that's used mainly to relieve mild to moderate pain. It works on the opioid receptor similar to opioid medications, but unlike opioids, it also works on other brain receptors.

Tramadol isn't a true opioid, but the drug isn't completely free of risks. Because it has the potential for abuse and it causes side effects similar to opioids, it's generally viewed as a narcotic. The most common side effects from the medication include dizziness, sedation, headache, nausea, constipation and seizures. Tramadol is also available in an extended-release form and in combination with acetaminophen. The combination drug is called Ultracet.

Topical medications

Topical medications are products that are applied to the skin to help relieve pain. These drugs act on the surface of your body or are absorbed locally through the skin where they may help relieve nerve pain and inflammation just below the skin's surface.

Local anesthetics

Local anesthetics inhibit pain signals along nerves at the site where the

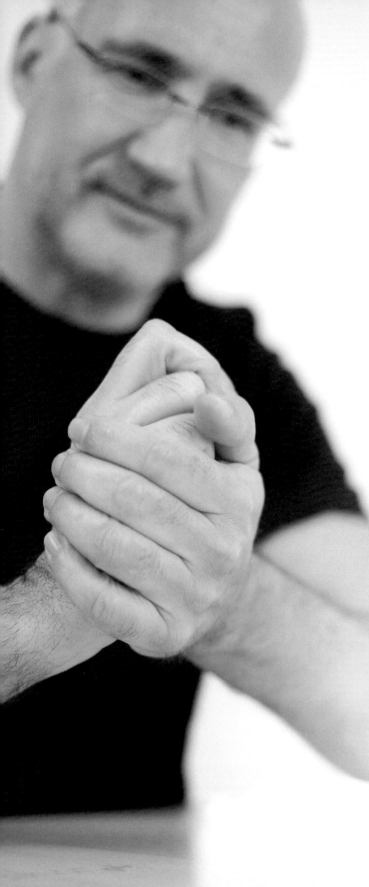

medication is applied. They're sold as patches, gels and creams.

Lidocaine patch

A lidocaine patch (Lidoderm) may be prescribed for relief of pain associated with postherpetic neuralgia and nerve pain. It's best used for pain that's localized to a specific site than for generalized pain. Redness and swelling may occur where the patch is applied.

Nonprescription products

There are several topical medications available without a prescription for pain relief. They include lidocaine (LMX4, Topicaine), benzocaine (Lanacane) and pramoxine (Prax, Itch-X).

Other analgesics

Other topical medications used to treat pain include the following:

Ketamine-amitriptyline cream

This product is a combination of the medications ketamine and amitriptyline. The cream is used most often for nerve-related (neuropathic) pain, including pain and tingling in the feet and hands (peripheral neuropathy) associated with diabetes. It's available only by prescription.

Capsaicin

This nonprescription drug is made from the seeds of hot chili peppers. It's thought to work by depleting nerve cells of a chemical called substance P, which has a role in transmitting pain messages.

You rub capsaicin (Capzasin-P, Zostrix) on your skin, typically three or five times a day. It usually takes up to two weeks before you begin to feel noticeable pain relief. Some people find capsaicin effective for temporary relief of arthritic pain in joints close to your skin's surface, such as your fingers, knees and elbows. It may also help relieve pain after shingles (postherpetic neuralgia). However, it can temporarily irritate your skin and produce a burning sensation, which is painful in and of itself.

Trolamine salicylate

Medications such as Aspercreme and Sportscreme contain a chemical that's similar to aspirin called trolamine salicylate. This chemical decreases the ability of nerve endings in the skin to sense pain. The Food and Drug Administration (FDA) lists products containing trolamine salicylate as safe, but not necessarily effective for pain relief. They're available without a prescription.

Counterirritant products

These nonprescription preparations (Bengay, Icy Hot) stimulate nerve endings in the skin to produce feelings of cold, warmth or itching. These responses, which may be mildly painful, counter more intense pain sensations.

Counterirritant products may relieve occasional, mild muscle aches and joint pain — simple strains and sprains — but they're generally not effective for most forms of chronic pain. In addition, they typically require frequent applications, and some products have a medicinal smell.

Other pain medications

Additional medications commonly used to treat chronic pain include drugs developed for other conditions, which have been found to be effective in relieving some types of pain.

Tricyclic antidepressants

Tricyclic antidepressants are a class of antidepressants that may be used to treat chronic pain. In addition to relieving symptoms of depression, tricyclic antidepressants interfere with certain chemical processes that cause you to feel pain. The drugs appear to strengthen the system that inhibits, or blocks, pain messages.

Tricyclic antidepressants commonly used to manage pain include:

- Amitriptyline
- Desipramine (Norpramin)
- Doxepin (Silenor)
- Imipramine (Tofranil)
- Nortriptyline (Pamelor)

Antidepressants don't cause dependence or addiction. However, tricyclic antidepressants can make you drowsy. Therefore, it's generally recommended that you take the medication in the evening before bed. In addition, these drugs may cause dry mouth, blurred vision, constipation, difficulty with urination, weight gain, changes in blood pressure and confusion.

Side effects usually begin soon after you start taking the medication or your dose is increased, but pain relief may not occur for several weeks. Tricyclic antidepressants can also interfere with the manner and rate at which the heart produces electrical impulses.

To reduce or prevent these symptoms, your doctor will likely start you off at a low dose and slowly increase the amount. Most people are able to take tricyclic antidepressants, particularly in low doses, with only mild side effects.

If your doctor prescribes a tricyclic antidepressant, he or she is likely using it to treat your pain, not depression. Higher doses of the medication are needed to treat depression, and there now are newer and more effective drugs for managing depression.

Serotonin and norepinephrine reuptake inhibitors (SNRIs)

This class of medications includes the drugs duloxetine (Cymbalta), venlafaxine (Effexor XR) and desvenlafaxine (Pristiq). Of these SNRI medications, only duloxetine has been approved by the FDA in the treatment of chronic pain. Duloxetine is an antidepressant that's sometimes prescribed to relieve pain caused by nerve damage in people with diabetes (diabetic neuropathy). The drug is thought to control pain by enhancing nerve signals within the central nervous system that naturally inhibit pain messages. Possible side effects include constipation, dizziness,

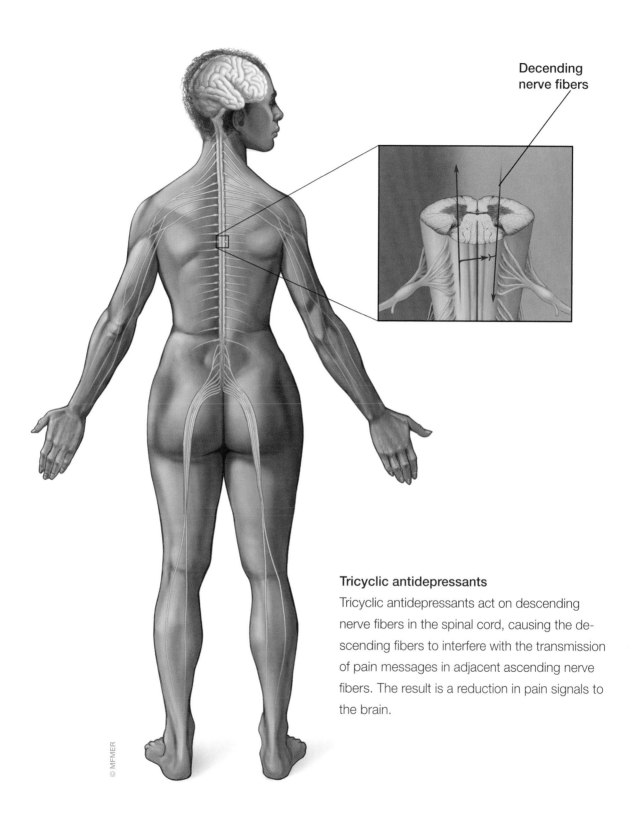

Decending nerve fibers

Tricyclic antidepressants

Tricyclic antidepressants act on descending nerve fibers in the spinal cord, causing the descending fibers to interfere with the transmission of pain messages in adjacent ascending nerve fibers. The result is a reduction in pain signals to the brain.

© MFMER

drowsiness, sleep problems, nausea and loss of appetite.

Anti-seizure medications

Several drugs developed primarily to control or reduce epileptic seizures have been found to help certain pain conditions, primarily the stabbing or shooting pain resulting from nerve damage. The drugs seem to work by quieting damaged nerves to slow or prevent uncontrolled pain signals.

Anti-seizure medications that may be used to treat chronic pain include:

- Carbamazepine (Carbatrol, Tegretol)
- Divalproex (Depakote)
- Gabapentin (Gralise, Neurontin)
- Lamotrigine (Lamictal)
- Phenytoin (Dilantin)
- Oxcarbazepine (Trileptal, Oxtellar XR)
- Pregabalin (Lyrica)
- Topiramate (Topamax)

These medications can cause dizziness, drowsiness, nausea, lack of balance and coordination, short-term memory disturbance, and weight gain or weight loss. More severe but less common side effects include skin, blood and liver disorders. To reduce your risk of side effects, your doctor will likely start you off on a small amount of the drug and gradually increase the dose.

Emotional symptoms

In addition to relieving your pain, there are other reasons that your doctor may prescribe medication. The intent of these drugs isn't direct relief of your pain, but relief of other troubling symptoms that can contribute to chronic pain. This is important because when you're not bothered by other symptoms, you can direct more of your energy toward your daily activities.

Depression and anxiety

Depression and anxiety are common among people with chronic pain. Relief from these conditions can have a significant effect on your ability to manage your pain. That's because as you begin to feel better — more energetic and more in control — your pain seems more tolerable and manageable.

Experts believe depression results from an imbalance in certain brain chemicals (neurotransmitters) that affect your

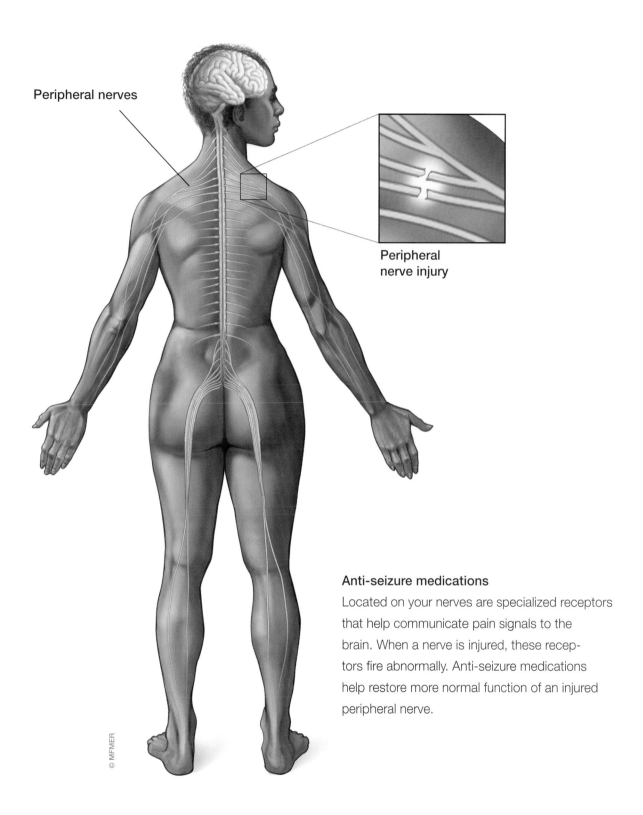

Peripheral nerves

Peripheral
nerve injury

Anti-seizure medications

Located on your nerves are specialized receptors that help communicate pain signals to the brain. When a nerve is injured, these receptors fire abnormally. Anti-seizure medications help restore more normal function of an injured peripheral nerve.

© MFMER

Buying medications online: The do's and don'ts

Ordering prescription drugs online can save you time and sometimes even money. But you must be careful. Questionable online pharmacies may ship expired drugs or those that haven't been stored properly. Others don't require a prescription or check for drug interactions. To safeguard your health and finances, remember these simple do's and don'ts.

Do:
- **Consult your doctor.** Your doctor can determine if it's OK to purchase your medication from an online site and also provide advice on cautions to be aware of, should you decide to do so.
- **Use a licensed pharmacy.** The National Association of Boards of Pharmacy can tell you whether a particular online pharmacy is licensed and in good standing.
- **Insist on access to a registered pharmacist.** Reputable sites offer toll-free access to registered pharmacists who can help answer your medication questions.

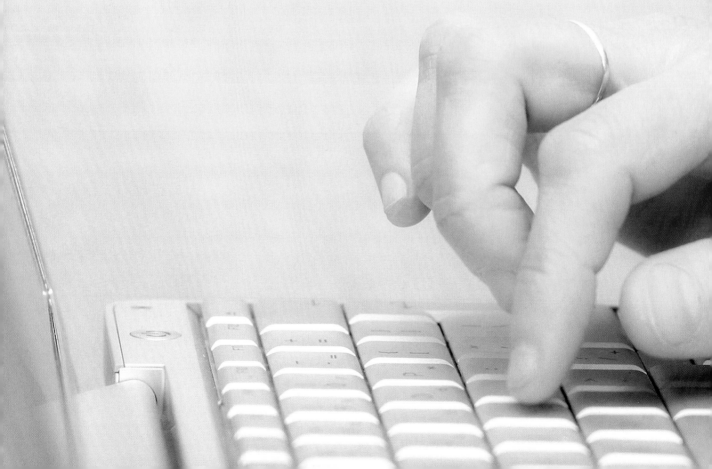

- **Read the privacy and security policies.** Before placing an order, be confident that your credit card number, personal health information and other personally identifiable information will be protected.
- **Be cautious of sites based in foreign countries.** Legitimate international sites exist. But there are risks. The medication may not be held to the same rigorous safety standards as in the United States.

Don't:
- **Use a site that bypasses prescriptions.** Only your doctor can safely prescribe medication.
- **Purchase medication that's not approved by the Food and Drug Administration.** Taking an inappropriate or unsafe drug may have life-threatening consequences.
- **Succumb to false claims.** Don't buy medication from sites that advertise "miracle cures" or those that use impressive terminology to disguise a lack of good science.

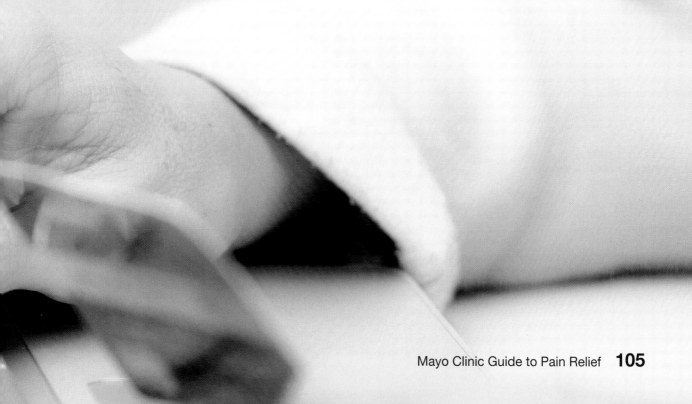

mood and emotions. The condition is often treated with medications that increase production of these chemicals. Anxiety is also thought to result from a combination of biochemical changes, and is treated with many of the same medications as depression.

In addition to tricyclic antidepressants and SNRIs, discussed earlier, other types of medications used to treat depression and anxiety include:

Selective serotonin reuptake inhibitors (SSRIs)

These medications have become a first line treatment for depression and anxiety because they produce few serious side effects. The drugs influence the activity of certain brain chemicals, helping nerve cells in your brain send and receive messages. SSRIs include the medications:

- Citalopram (Celexa)
- Escitalopram (Lexapro)
- Fluoxetine (Prozac, Sarafem)
- Paroxetine (Paxil)
- Sertraline (Zoloft)

SSRIs don't work immediately. It may take up to eight weeks before you experience the full effects of the drugs. They can also cause some side effects. Several people on SSRIs report sexual side effects. Once you stop taking the drug, sexual problems usually go away. Other side effects may include headache, dizziness, nausea and diarrhea.

Other antidepressants

These medications work similarly to SSRIs, but they affect different brain chemicals:

- Bupropion (Wellbutrin)
- Mirtazapine (Remeron)
- Venlafaxine (Effexor XR)

Anxiolytics

Anxiolytics are a form of benzodiazepines that reduce feelings of anxiety and often cause sedation. They include the medications:

- Alprazolam (Niravam, Xanax)
- Clonazepam (Klonopin)
- Diazepam (Valium)
- Lorazepam (Ativan)

Anxiolytics can become habit-forming if you take them for more than a few weeks. Your doctor may prescribe the medication for only a short time to get you through an anxious period.

Buspirone

This is an anti-anxiety medication that works by stimulating serotonin receptors on nerves, altering the chemical messages that nerves transmit to each other. Unlike some other anti-anxiety medications, buspirone doesn't cause sedation. However, it takes a couple of weeks for the effects of the drug to become noticeable.

Buspirone is most effective for mild to moderate anxiety symptoms. Side effects may include dizziness, headache, nausea and insomnia.

Sleep troubles

Pain affects sleep. If you're in pain, you may have trouble falling asleep or your pain may wake you up at night and you may not be able to get back to sleep. Just the opposite, the medication you're taking for your pain may make you drowsy and cause too much sleep.

A good night's sleep is important because it can help you better cope with your pain by renewing your energy level and improving your mood. The best treatment for improving sleep is to improve your sleep habits (see page 202). Medications to help promote sleep may be prescribed for a short period until your change in habits have had time to become effective.

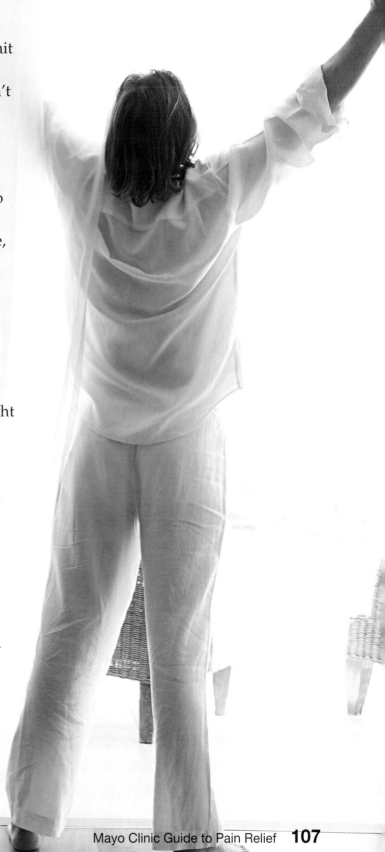

Antidepressants

Drowsiness is a common side effect of some antidepressants. When taken at night before bed, the drugs may help you sleep better — in addition to controlling pain and depression. The antidepressant trazodone (Desyrel) is commonly prescribed to help improve sleep.

Sedatives

Sedatives help promote sleep, but they may affect your alertness during the day, even when you don't feel drowsy. They can also cloud your thinking, impair your balance and affect your ability to drive. If taken for more than just a short period, some sedatives may also cause dependency or addiction.

Sedatives can be divided into two broad categories — benzodiazepines and nonbenzodiazepines. Benzodiazepines are an older class of sleeping pills. They're more likely to cause headache and drowsiness in the morning, and they can be habit-forming. Benzodiazepines include:

- Estazolam
- Temazepam (Restoril)
- Triazolam (Halcion)

Nonbenzodiazepines induce sleep by quieting the nervous system.

Commonly prescribed nonbenzodiazepines include:

- Eszopiclone (Lunesta)
- Zaleplon (Sonata)
- Zolpidem (Ambien)

It's important to remember that sleeping pills are a temporary solution for your sleep problems while other efforts to improve your sleep have time to work. They should be used for only a few nights at a time. Many sedatives have been found to promote activities during sleep including sleepwalking, sleep-eating and sleep-driving, in which people get out of bed and perform tasks or activities during the night that they have no recollection of in the morning.

Other conditions

Sometimes, chronic pain is associated with other physical conditions that also need to be addressed in order for pain relief treatments to be effective.

Muscle spasms

If your pain is accompanied by muscle spasms, your doctor may recommend a muscle relaxant to control the spasms. Muscle relaxants are best used on a short-term, as-needed basis — a period of three to five days — because they can cause side effects. For example, the drugs can cloud your thinking and leave you drowsy and dizzy, especially when taken in combination with an opioid. Muscle relaxants include these prescription drugs:

- Carisoprodol (Soma)
- Cyclobenzaprine (Amrix)
- Methocarbamol (Robaxin)
- Orphenadrine (Norflex)
- Tizanidine (Zanaflex)

Inflammation

If your pain is related to rheumatoid arthritis or another inflammatory condition, your doctor may prescribe oral anti-inflammatory medications, including NSAIDs and steroids. These drugs are used both to ease the pain and to reduce inflammation that may damage your joints.

If you have an acutely inflamed joint, an NSAID may not be effective and your doctor may prescribe an oral corticosteroid. Corticosteroids may be used short term or, in some cases, long term to manage a more serious problem. Widely used corticosteroids include the oral drugs hydrocortisone and prednisone.

Weighing the benefits and risks

There's no question that medications play an important role in the treatment of chronic pain, but they should be used judiciously — weighing the benefits of a particular drug against its potential for serious side effects. Medication is generally considered to be of benefit if it can result in less pain, improved function and a return to everyday activities, while causing only minimal side effects.

Some people learn to manage their pain without drugs. Medication may be used initially while a comprehensive treatment plan is developed and put in place, but medication may not be necessary long term. These individuals may still have some pain, but they're able to function well despite the pain.

As you consider the role of medications in controlling your pain it's important to remember that each person is different and not all people respond in the same manner to various medications. A drug that works for one person may not for you. Likewise, a drug that you find helpful may be of little benefit to someone else.

In addition, some people have difficulty taking pain medication in the manner that's prescribed, leading to possible abuse. Though most people do not abuse prescription medications, the problem is increasing, especially among young people. If your doctor feels that use of pain medications could become a problem, he or she may be reluctant to prescribe them.

The main thing to remember is not to make judgments based simply on what you read or hear. The best place to get advice about the use of medications is from your doctor or another health care professional who is helping you manage your pain.

Prescription drug abuse

An issue that cannot be overlooked when prescription medications are involved — especially those used to control pain — is that of prescription drug abuse. Prescription drug abuse is the use of a prescription medication in a way not intended by the doctor who prescribed it. This includes taking more of a medication than prescribed for your pain and taking a drug for the feelings you get from it, not because you need it to relieve pain or other symptoms.

Prescription drug abuse includes everything from taking a friend's prescription painkiller for a backache to snorting or injecting ground-up pills to get high. Drug abuse may become ongoing and compulsive, despite the negative consequences.

The Centers for Disease Control and Prevention (CDC) reports that drug overdose death rates in the United States have more than tripled in recent years and have never been higher. According to the most recent figures available, more than 36,000 people die from drug overdoses annually, and most of the deaths are caused by prescription drugs.

Prescription drug abuse can affect all age groups. Misuse of medications is a growing problem in older adults. Having multiple health problems and taking multiple drugs can put seniors at risk of misusing drugs or becoming

Signs and symptoms of prescription drug abuse

Opioid painkillers	Sedatives and anti-anxiety medications	Stimulants
Constipation	Drowsiness	Weight loss
Depression	Confusion	Agitation
Low blood pressure	Unsteady walking	Irritability
Decreased breathing rate	Poor judgment	Insomnia
Confusion	Involuntary, rapid eye movement	High blood pressure
Sweating	Dizziness	Irregular heartbeat
Poor coordination		Restlessness
		Impulsive behavior

addicted to them, especially when they combine drugs with alcohol. But prescription drug abuse is most common in young people. The prescription drugs most often abused include painkillers, sedatives, anti-anxiety medications and stimulants.

Symptoms

Early identification of drug abuse and early intervention may prevent the problem from turning into an addiction. Because of their mind-altering properties, the most commonly abused prescription drugs are:

- **Opioids.** These medications taken to treat pain include oxycodone (OxyContin) and medications containing hydrocodone (Lortab).

- **Anti-anxiety medications and sedatives.** This group of drugs includes medications such as alprazolam (Niravam, Xanax) and diazepam (Valium), and hypnotics such as zolpidem (Ambien), used to treat anxiety and sleep disorders.
- **Stimulants.** Stimulants such as methylphenidate (Ritalin) are taken to treat ADHD and certain sleep disorders.

Signs and symptoms of prescription drug abuse depend on the particular drug (see the chart above). Other signs of abuse include:

- Stealing, forging or selling prescriptions
- Taking higher doses than prescribed
- Excessive mood swings or hostility
- Increase or decrease in sleep

- Poor decision-making
- Appearing to be high, unusually energetic or revved up, or sedated
- Continually "losing" prescriptions, so more prescriptions must be written
- Seeking prescriptions from more than one doctor

Causes

Teens and adults abuse prescription drugs for a number of reasons, including:

- To feel good or get high
- To relax or relieve tension
- To reduce appetite or increase alertness
- To experiment with the mental effects of the substance
- To maintain an addiction and prevent withdrawal
- To be accepted by peers (peer pressure) or to be social
- To try to improve concentration and academic or work performance

Risk factors

Many people fear that they may become addicted to medications prescribed for legitimate medical conditions, such as painkillers prescribed after surgery.

However, people who take potentially addictive drugs as prescribed rarely abuse them or become addicted.

Risk factors for prescription drug abuse include:

- Past or present addictions to other substances, including alcohol
- Younger age, specifically the teens or early 20s
- Certain pre-existing psychiatric conditions
- Exposure to peer pressure or a social environment where there's drug use
- Easier access to prescription drugs, such as working in a health care setting
- Lack of knowledge about prescription drugs

Complications

Abusing prescription drugs can cause a number of problems. Misuse of medications can be especially dangerous when the drugs are taken in high doses, combined with certain prescription or over-the-counter medications, or taken with alcohol or illegal drugs.

- Misuse of opioids can cause an increased risk of choking, low blood pressure, a slowed breathing rate and potential for breathing to stop, or a coma.

- Misuse of sedatives or anti-anxiety medications can cause memory problems, low blood pressure and slowed breathing. An overdose can cause coma or death.
- Misuse of stimulants can cause dangerously high body temperature, heart problems, high blood pressure, seizures or tremors, hallucinations, aggressiveness, and paranoia.

Addiction

Because commonly abused prescription drugs activate the brain's reward center, it's possible to become addicted to them. People who are addicted continue to use a drug even when that drug makes their lives worse — just like people addicted to nicotine continue smoking cigarettes even when it harms their health and they want to quit.

Other consequences

Other potential consequences include engaging in risky behaviors because of poor judgment, using illegal drugs, being involved in a crime, having a motor vehicle accident, performing poorly in school or at work, and experiencing increased difficulties with relationships.

When to see a doctor

Talk to your doctor if you think you may have a drug abuse problem. You may feel embarrassed to talk to your doctor about it — but remember that medical professionals are trained to help you, not judge you. Identifying prescription drug abuse as soon as possible is important. It's easier to tackle the problem early before it becomes an addiction and leads to more serious problems.

Your primary care doctor may be able to help you overcome a prescription drug abuse problem. However, if you have an addiction, your doctor may refer you to an addiction specialist or to a facility that specializes in helping people withdraw from drugs.

Treatment

Treatment options for prescription drug abuse vary, but counseling, also called talk therapy or psychotherapy, is typically a key part of treatment.

Counseling. Counseling — whether it's individual, group or family counseling — can help determine what factors may have led to the abuse, such as an underlying mental health problem or relationship problems. Counseling can also help you learn the skills needed to resist cravings, avoid abuse of drugs and help prevent recurrence of prescription drug problems. Through counseling, you can learn strategies for developing positive relationships and identify ways to become involved in healthy activities that aren't related to drugs.

Medications. Detoxification is sometimes part of treatment. Drug withdrawal can be dangerous and should be done under a doctor's care. Depending on the type of drug taken, it may take weeks or even months to slowly taper off the medication. It can take a while for your body to adjust to low doses of the drug and then get used to taking no medication at all. You may need other types of medications to deal with withdrawal symptoms, such as sleep, appetite and mood disturbances.

Helping a loved one

It can be difficult to approach a loved one about prescription drug abuse. Denial and anger are common reactions, and you may be concerned

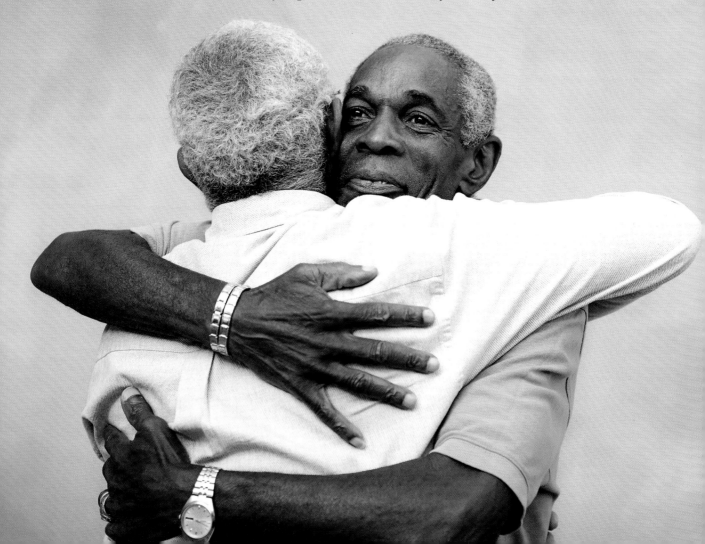

about creating conflict or damaging your relationship with that person. Be understanding and patient. Let the person know that you care about his or her well-being. Encourage your loved one to be honest about drug use and to accept help if needed. A person is more likely to respond to feedback from someone they trust. If the problem continues, further intervention may be necessary.

Intervention

It can be challenging to help a loved one struggling with drug problems or other destructive behavior. People who struggle with addictive behaviors are often in denial about their situation or are unwilling to seek treatment, and they don't recognize the negative effects their behavior has on themselves and others. An intervention can motivate someone to seek help for addictive behaviors.

An intervention is a carefully planned process involving family and friends and others who care about a person struggling with addiction. Consulting an intervention professional (interventionist), an addiction specialist, psychologist or mental health counselor can help you organize an effective intervention. This is an opportunity to confront the person about the consequences of addiction and ask him or her to accept treatment. Think of an intervention as giving your loved one a clear opportunity to make changes before things get really bad.

Preventing abuse in teens

Young people are at especially high risk of prescription drug abuse. To help prevent your teen from abusing prescription medications, follow these steps:

- **Discuss the dangers.** Emphasize to your teen that just because drugs are prescribed by a doctor, it doesn't mean they're safe — especially if they were prescribed to someone else or if your child is already taking other prescription medications.
- **Set rules about medication use.** Let your teen know that it's not OK to share medications with others — or to take medications prescribed for others. Emphasize the importance of taking the prescribed dose of medication and talking with the doctor before making changes.
- **Keep your prescription drugs safe.** Keep your medications and those of other family members locked in a medicine cabinet and keep track of quantities. If you seem to be running out of a medication sooner

than you should be, that could be a
red flag. Figure out why.

- **Make sure your teen isn't ordering
drugs online.** Some websites sell
counterfeit and dangerous drugs
that may not require a prescription.
- **Properly dispose of medications.**
Check the label or patient information guide for disposal instructions.
You can ask your pharmacist or local
trash and recycling service if there's
a medicine take-back program that
accepts unused medications. If not,
put unused drugs in your household
trash. But before throwing them out,
remove them from the container and
mix them in a sealed plastic bag with
used coffee grounds, used kitty litter
or another undesirable substance.
Before tossing the container, remove
the label and cross out identifying
information.

Chapter 8

Injections, stimulators and pumps

When it comes to methods to relieve pain, the first thing most people think of is medication. However, there are several ways to treat chronic pain beyond oral medications. Options range from using needles to inject medication at or near the site of the pain, to implanting pain-relieving devices in your body, such as nerve stimulators and medication pumps. Depending on the type of pain you have and its severity, one of these approaches may work for you.

Injection therapy

Instead of prescribing pills to control the pain, your doctor might inject medication at or near the pain site to see if it can provide pain relief. Injections generally don't cure pain, but they may help you through an initial period of intense pain or a flare-up of severe pain.

Injections are most effective for joint, muscle or nerve pain that's confined to a specific location. The type of drug injected may be an anesthetic to control the pain, a steroid to reduce inflammation or a combination of the two.

One benefit of injections is that the medication works primarily, but not exclusively, in a limited part of your body. By targeting a specific area, injections may reduce the amount of medication needed and the possible side effects.

In addition to providing pain relief, injections are sometimes used to help diagnose the cause of your pain. Suppose, for example, that a small amount of anesthetic injected at a specific location relieves your pain. This indicates that a particular joint, muscle or nerve may be the source of the pain. Once your doctor knows the pain source, it's possible he or she can find more effective methods to treat it.

In deciding whether injections may be right for you, keep in mind that you'll have to visit your doctor's office for each procedure. In addition, the site of the injection and the type of medication used can limit how often you receive an injection. For instance, injected steroids may cause adverse side effects that become worse with frequent use. This is why doctors generally limit the number of injections that you can have, and why it's important to make your doctor aware of any injections you've received for pain within the last year.

Injections are seldom used by themselves to treat chronic pain. They're generally most effective when given in conjunction with a program that also includes physical therapy. Injections can make the therapy more comfortable.

The types of injections used to treat chronic pain can be divided into three broad categories: peripheral joint and nerve injections, soft tissue injections and spinal injections.

Peripheral joint and nerve injections

Peripheral injections are used to reduce pain in large, weight-bearing joints and in major peripheral nerves. Your peripheral nerves extend from your spinal cord to your arms, hands, legs and feet.

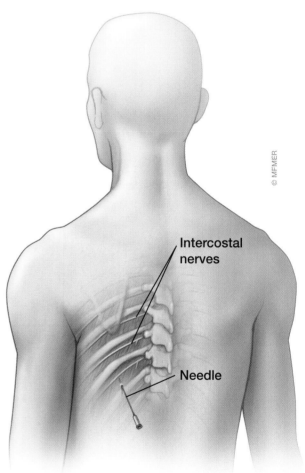

Intercostal injection

An intercostal injection blocks the transmission of pain signals in the intercostal nerves, which originate in the spinal cord and run under the ribs.

Your peripheral joints include your hip and knee joints, and other large joints such as your shoulder and elbow joints. When these joints become inflamed and painful, your doctor may inject medications into them to ease your discomfort. Peripheral joint injections can provide immediate pain relief, giving other methods to control the pain, such as physical therapy or oral medications, time to work.

Peripheral nerve injections work in the same way, but instead of the medication being injected into a joint, it's injected around a specific group of nerves. This temporarily prevents pain messages traveling along that nerve pathway from reaching your brain.

In addition to helping manage pain, peripheral nerve injections are also used to help diagnose the source of pain. If a medication injected near a specific nerve eliminates or significantly reduces your pain, doctors know that nerve is likely the source of your pain.

Commonly targeted nerves include the following:

Intercostal nerves. These nerves lie between the ribs. An intercostal injection may be used to help control pain from an injured nerve in the rib area.

Occipital nerves. The occipital nerves provide sensation to the back of the neck and head. An occipital injection is given at the base of the skull or back of the neck. It may be used in the diagnosis or treatment of conditions such as headache or chronic jaw pain.

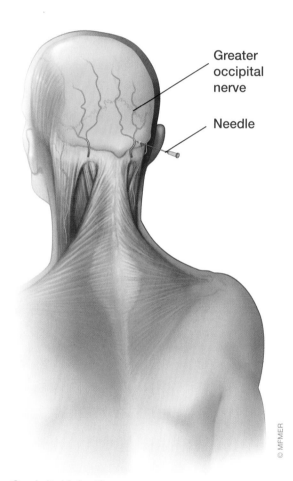

Occipital injection

An occipital injection is performed at the base of the skull, blocking transmission of signals from the occipital nerve. The occipital nerves originate in the upper (cervical) spine.

Injections in the knee joint

For a number of years, a compound containing derivatives of hyaluronic acid — commonly known by the brand names Synvisc and Hyalgan — has been injected into knee joints to help treat osteoarthritis of the knee.

Hyaluronic acid is a lubricating substance found in normal joint fluid. In people with osteoarthritis, hyaluronic acid often thins out and there isn't enough of the acid to provide adequate protection to the joint. In an attempt to improve lubrication and joint mobility, a compound containing hyaluronic acid is injected into the knee joint in a series of shots.

There's some controversy as to whether these injections are effective. Some studies and reviews suggest that the injections aren't very effective. They may help some people initially, but the benefits generally don't last beyond six months. There's also no evidence they slow progression of the disease.

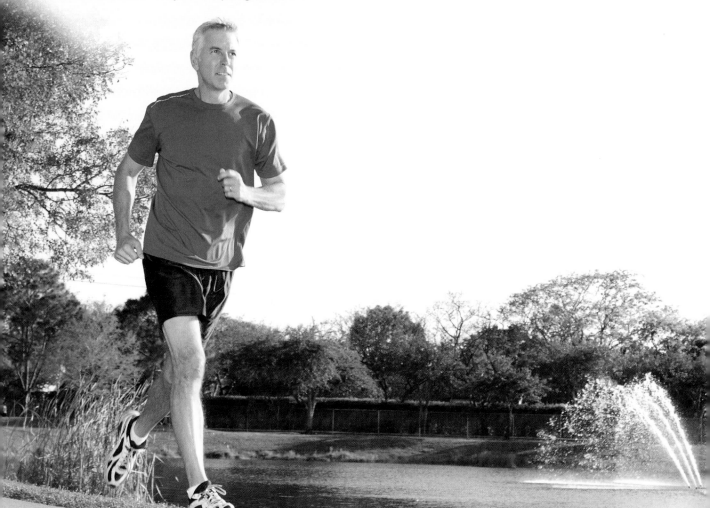

Large peripheral nerves. With this type of injection, medication is placed in the area surrounding a large peripheral nerve, such as the femoral nerve, the major nerve that runs from your spine down each of your legs. These types of injections may be used to help relieve leg or arm pain resulting from damage to or pressure on a large peripheral nerve.

Medications

The most common types of medication used in peripheral joint and nerve injections are local anesthetics and steroid medications. The drugs may be given separately or combined into one shot:

Local anesthetic. A local anesthetic is used to temporarily numb a painful area. It works by interfering with, or blocking, pain pathways to the brain. The result is less pain in that area for a short period. You may also experience reduced feeling at the injection site because the nerves have been numbed.

Steroid. Long-acting injected steroid medications help decrease pain by reducing inflammation in joints and around nerves. Steroids may be injected into one or several affected areas of your body, such as the shoulder, elbow, hip or knee. In the short term, corticosteroids can make you feel dramatically

better and they may provide pain relief for two to three months. But when used for many months or years, they may cause serious side effects, such as weakened cartilage and ligaments, easy bruising, thinning of bones, cataracts, weight gain, a round face, diabetes, high blood pressure, and a decreased ability to heal wounds and fight infections.

Soft tissue injections

When a specific part of your body — such as a muscle or bursa — is inflamed and painful, an injection may be given directly into the surrounding soft tissue. There are two main types of soft tissue injections.

Trigger point injections. Trigger points are areas where your muscles and surrounding connective tissue are sensitive to touch. Trigger points are generally located in the upper and lower back muscles, but they may occur elsewhere (see page 122). Trigger point injections are used when your muscles are overly sensitive and are a source of pain. Depending on the medication used, trigger point injections may help reduce pain in a muscle, reduce inflammation or relax an overly sensitive muscle.

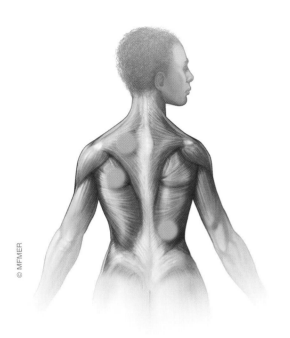

© MFMER

Trigger points

The areas highlighted in green are common trigger points. Medication may be injected in these areas to relieve pain in overly sensitive muscles.

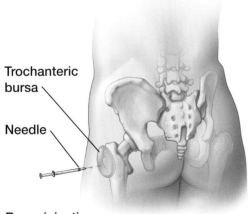

Trochanteric bursa

Needle

Bursa injection

A local anesthetic and steroid medication are injected into a bursa to reduce the pain and inflammation of bursitis.

Bursa injections. Bursae are tiny, fluid-filled sacs that lubricate and cushion pressure points between your bones and the tendons and muscles near your joints. You have more than 150 bursae in your body, which help you move without pain. When bursae become inflamed (bursitis), movement of or pressure on the affected joint becomes painful. Bursitis most often affects the shoulder, elbow or hip areas.

Medications

Medications used in soft tissue injections include:

Local anesthetic. A local anesthetic is used to provide immediate pain relief. Often an anesthetic is given in conjunction with a steroid medication, but sometimes an anesthetic may be given by itself.

Steroid. A corticosteroid medication is injected into soft tissue to help reduce inflammation, which ultimately results in reduced pain. It may take three to four days before the medication starts working. Reducing inflammation and pain allows for increased movement in the affected area. Effects may last from a few weeks to several months.

Botox. A type of toxin known as ona-botulinumtoxinA (Botox) is injected into one or more muscles that are causing pain. The toxin causes temporary paralysis of these muscles. Botox injections may be used if you have a condition caused by cramping muscles (dystonia), certain types of headaches or other disorders involving chronic muscle spasm. The amount of toxin used is very small. Its effects generally last about three months. Repeat injections are often needed.

Spinal injections

Spinal injections are used in situations in which chronic pain is thought to be associated with a spinal joint or nerve that's been damaged or is irritated or inflamed. A local anesthetic may be injected to numb the pain, a steroid medication given to reduce inflammation or a combination of both.

An injection directly into the spinal fluid is called an intrathecal (in-truh-THEE-kul) injection. This type of injection is the kind often used during surgery involving the abdomen or lower extremities. If the injection isn't into the spinal fluid, it's called an epidural injection. Epidurals are often used to relieve the pain of childbirth, and they may be given to relieve some types of back pain, such as sciatica.

In addition to treating pain, spinal injections can help diagnose the cause of pain. If medication placed in a certain location relieves the pain, doctors are able to focus on the pain source.

Spinal injections are performed with the guidance of fluoroscopy, an X-ray imaging procedure that allows the doctor or imaging specialist to view the spinal column as the needle containing the medication is inserted. For this procedure, you may be asked to lie facedown on the examining table or on your side.

There are several types of spinal injections. Some of the more common injections include:

Epidural. Epidural injections are the most common. In this procedure, a needle is inserted between the back bones into the epidural space that surrounds the spinal cord and spinal nerves (see page 124). Epidural injections may be given in the neck (cervical), midback (thoracic) and low back (lumbar) regions. The medication coats nerves in the location where it's injected, relieving pain.

Transforaminal epidural. In these injections, the needle containing medication is inserted into the epidural space

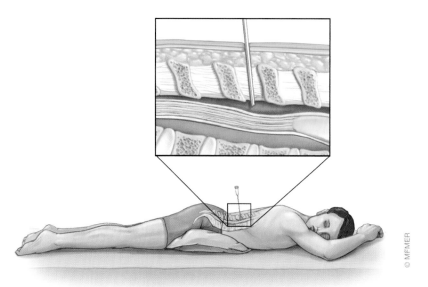

Epidural injection

An epidural injection is performed under X-ray guidance. A needle is positioned in the epidural space in the spinal column, and medications are injected to relieve the pain.

through the opening of an exiting nerve root. This technique allows the medication to be placed closer to a nerve root responsible for the pain than does the standard epidural approach.

Selective nerve root. In this type of injection, medication is placed around the nerve root after it leaves the spine. This type of injection is used mostly to diagnose a painful condition. It can help determine which nerve root is the predominant source of pain.

Facet joint. In this procedure, medication is injected into one or more facet joints — small, stabilizing joints located between and behind the spine's verte-

brae. The medication, typically a steroid, reduces inflammation and swelling within the joint that's causing pain.

Sympathetic block. With this type of injection, medication is inserted into nerve tissue that's part of the sympathetic nervous system. The sympathetic nerves are located in the back and neck on either side of the spine. Sympathetic blocks help reduce pain and swelling, as well as color and sweating changes in the legs and feet. The injections are used to treat conditions such as complex regional pain syndrome.

Celiac plexus block. A local anesthetic is injected into a group of nerves serving the body's abdominal organs (celiac plexus nerves). This block is done most often to treat chronic upper abdominal pain and pain from pancreatic cancer.

Sacroiliac joint. These types of injections are given in the sacroiliac joint, which is located in the buttock region.

They're used to treat a type of low back-buttock pain.

Piriformis muscle. A piriformis injection may be used in people experiencing impingement of the sciatic nerve as the nerve passes through the piriformis muscle, a muscle located behind the

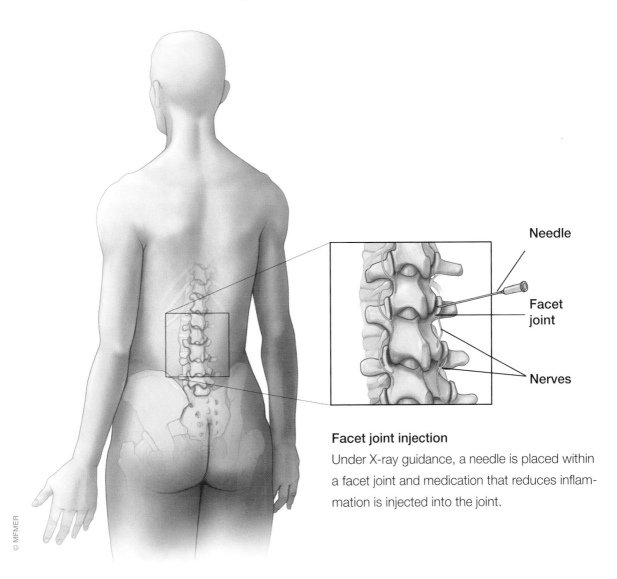

Facet joint injection
Under X-ray guidance, a needle is placed within a facet joint and medication that reduces inflammation is injected into the joint.

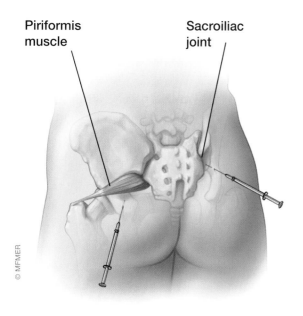

Piriformis muscle

Sacroiliac joint

© MFMER

Sacroiliac and piriformis injections
In these procedures, medication is injected into the sacroiliac joint or piriformis muscle to relieve low back or leg pain.

hip joint. Medication is injected into the muscle to help relieve the pain.

Discogram. This procedure is used to determine which disk or disks in your back are causing pain. A solution is injected into one or more disks in an attempt to re-create the pain by increasing pressure in the disk.

Radiofrequency ablation. A needle used in conjunction with nerve stimulation is placed near a painful nerve. Heat produced by radio waves (high-frequency energy) runs through the

needle to the nerve, heats up nerve tissue and disrupts pain signals coming from the tissue. The disruption blocks nerve signals to the brain. The procedure isn't a permanent treatment. The nerves often grow back, and the procedure may need to be repeated.

Nerve stimulators

Nerve stimulators are electronic devices that produce electrical signals to stimulate certain nerves, with the goal of reducing pain. They include transcutaneous electrical nerve stimulators (TENS), spinal cord stimulators and peripheral nerve stimulators.

TENS

For this type of nerve stimulation, electrodes are placed on your skin near the painful area. The electrodes are attached to a small, portable, battery-powered unit. The unit generates low-level, painless electric impulses that pass through your skin to underlying nerve fibers to modify your pain perception. You adjust settings on the TENS unit as needed to control the electric impulse level. You can wear the device at home or at work.

Exactly how TENS works isn't known. It may trigger the release of endorphins — chemicals in your body that have painkilling effects similar to the drug morphine. TENS treatment may also block nerve pathways that carry pain messages.

TENS generally works best for mild pain, and not all people who use the device benefit from it. Most often, TENS is combined with exercise and other pain treatments.

A similar treatment called percutaneous electrical nerve stimulation (PENS) is used in combination with acupuncture. Instead of transmitting the current through electrodes placed on top of your skin, PENS uses thin needles that penetrate your skin to just below its surface. Most people feel some sensation, but not pain, when the needles are inserted. Unlike TENS, percutaneous electrical nerve stimulation must be performed by a trained practitioner and cannot be used at home or at work.

Spinal cord and peripheral nerve stimulators

Spinal cord and peripheral nerve stimulators may be a treatment option for people who suffer from certain types of chronic pain conditions. These electronic devices aren't a cure for the pain. Rather, their objective is to reduce the pain to a more manageable level.

Spinal cord and peripheral nerve stimulators are most often used when traditional treatments for pain, such as medication or surgery, are ineffective, not feasible or they cause unwanted side effects.

During a short surgical procedure, a thin wire called a lead is placed in the space that surrounds the spinal cord and spinal nerves (epidural space) or alongside a large peripheral nerve — depending on the type and source of your pain. An electrical generator also is inserted under the skin. The lead is connected to the generator, and when the generator's power is turned on, electrical power is sent through the lead to an electrode — in the form a needle — attached at the other end.

The electrode stimulates nerve fibers at the location where you're experiencing pain. The hope is that the stimulation will alter the pain messages and replace them with more pleasant sensations (paresthesia). These sensations differ, but people often describe them as a tingling feeling.

Electrode or catheter

Drug infusion device or electrical generator placed beneath the skin

© MFMER

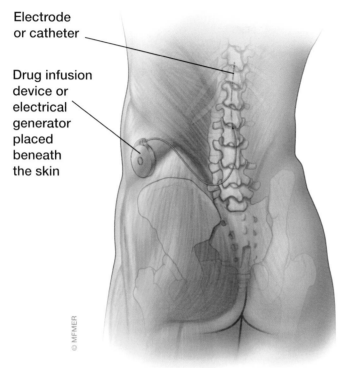

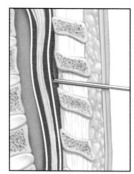

With a nerve stimulator, an electrode is placed in the epidural space within the spinal canal.

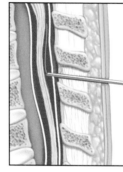

With a pain pump, medication is administered through a catheter to the intrathecal space in the spinal canal.

Nerve stimulators and pain pumps

Each of these procedures is performed under X-ray guidance. With both procedures, a needle is inserted into the correct location. In the case of a nerve stimulator, an electrode is then positioned in the epidural space and the needle is removed. With a pain pump, the needle is inserted into the intrathecal space and is removed once a catheter that administers the medication is positioned correctly.

There are different types of neuro-stimulation, and the type that's right for you depends on many factors, including the cause of your pain or neurological disorder, as well as its type and location. Recent improvements to spinal cord stimulators include rechargeable batteries. An external device held over the implanted unit recharges the battery, reducing the number of surgeries needed to replace worn-out batteries.

If you're a candidate for spinal cord or peripheral nerve stimulation, you'll likely undergo a stimulation trial to find out how well you respond to the therapy before you commit to surgery to fully implant the system. For some people the sensation emitted by the stimulator isn't pleasant nor does it relieve the pain.

Medication pumps

Commonly referred to as medication pumps or pain pumps, the technical term for these devices is intrathecal drug delivery systems. They deliver pain medication directly to the fluid that surrounds the spinal cord (cerebrospinal fluid).

Medication pumps are most often used to treat cancer pain and chronic pain that doesn't respond to other types of treatment. This may include pain resulting from nerve damage or illness and pain associated with muscle spasm resulting from injury to the spinal cord.

A medication pump consists of a small flexible catheter that's placed in the spinal fluid. The catheter is connected to a drug infusion pump that's implanted into your lower abdomen. The medication is placed into the pump via a small covered opening (port) in the top of the pump.

A computerized program tells the pump how much of the medication you are to receive, dispensing the drug at a set rate. The medication may be an opioid (narcotic) or a local anesthetic, a muscle relaxant, or other medication. The muscle relaxant baclofen (Lioresal) or the new analgesic medication ziconotide (Prialt) may be used. Ziconotide was developed specifically for use in medication pumps.

This method of drug delivery may reduce your pain and cause fewer side effects than do oral pain medications. This is because less medication may be needed when the medication is delivered directly to pain receptors in the spinal cord.

Similar to a spinal cord stimulator, your doctor will likely recommend that you first undergo a screening trial before the device is permanently implanted to see if the treatment will help you.

You may have to restrict some activities while using a medication pump. That's because the pain medication being dispensed may produce numbness, which can reduce your ability to sense pressure and temperature changes, in addition to pain. The numbness often decreases with time, but it may not go away entirely. Another drawback of these devices is that they're expensive.

Choosing the right treatment

The procedures and technologies described in this chapter offer a variety of treatment options. Keep in mind that these options don't exclude one another. For instance, someone with chronic pain may receive physical therapy as well as use a spinal cord stimulator.

Selecting a technology that's best for you involves consideration of several factors. Be sure to discuss the following issues — as well as any other questions you have — with your doctor.

Your expectations. Stimulators and medication pumps represent the latest in pain management technology. However, no technology offers total pain relief. Technology can lessen your discomfort, but you'll probably continue to feel some pain. A reasonable goal is to reduce your pain by 50 percent.

It's important to remember that injections and more invasive treatments, such as stimulators, are most effective when they're used with other therapies. They're also just one option to consider. For many pain syndromes, good habits such as eating well and getting regular exercise are very important and can't be overlooked.

Your treatment history. Before prescribing devices such as implantable stimulators and pumps, your doctor may first try a variety of other treatments, such as oral medication, physical therapy, exercise and counseling. Stimulators and pumps are generally recommended only after you've tried less invasive and less expensive options. Knowing how you've responded to pain treatments in the past can help predict how well a new technology may work for you.

Your medical evaluation. In addition to standard tests, such as checking your blood pressure and heart rate, your doctor may require that you have a psychological evaluation. A psychological evaluation recognizes that your mind and body are connected. The success of any medical treatment may depend in part on your feelings about the treatment as well as how you cope with pain on a day-to-day basis.

Medical risks and side effects. Surgery is needed to implant a device in your body, and surgery carries some risk. In addition, pain medications have side effects — a factor to consider with injections or any device that delivers medication.

Your range of pain. When chronic pain is localized in a particular area of your body, injections or peripheral nerve stimulation may be the best option. For pain that spreads over a larger region of your body, a spinal cord stimulator or medication pump might be more useful. But again, no technology offers total pain relief.

Your comfort level. Like any piece of technology, pumps and stimula- tors require general maintenance and troubleshooting. Most spinal cord stimulators in use today have a rechargeable battery that you need to recharge. Pump batteries aren't rechargeable and must be changed from time to time. Pumps must also be refilled with medication. Be sure that you fully understand all that's involved in using a pump or stimulator.

Where you live and travel. If your medication pump runs out of medication

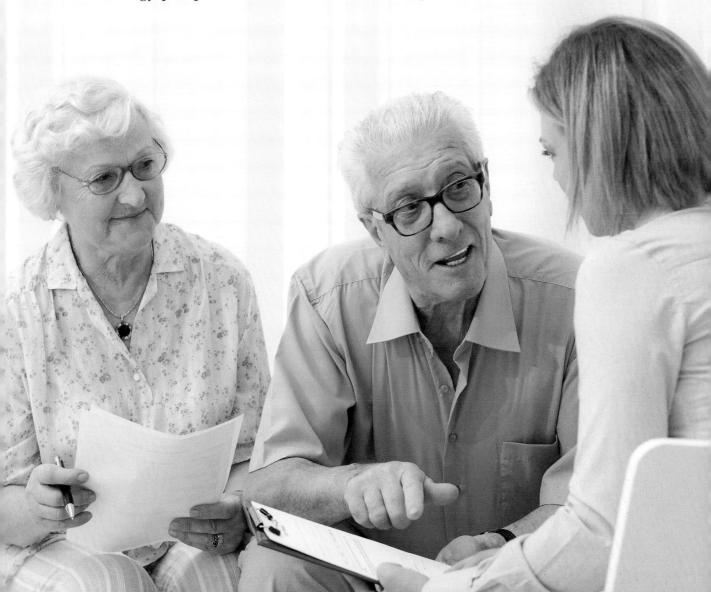

or malfunctions, you may experience withdrawal symptoms, changes in blood pressure or other complications. During such a situation, you'll need to find to a doctor comfortable in managing such a device. This may be a factor in determining the best treatment for you.

Insurance coverage. Most medical insurers will cover the cost of pain relief technology, but you'll need to work with your doctor and insurance company in order to satisfy requirements for coverage.

Chapter 9

Pain specialists and rehabilitation centers

Major life changes sometimes require personal guidance. Learning how to manage chronic pain is one instance where one-on-one help may make a difference. If you feel that you might benefit from more individualized care, you may want to see an individual who specializes in pain medicine. Or, perhaps, your primary care doctor has recommended that you see a pain specialist.

Pain specialists, or pain medicine doctors, can help diagnose the cause of your pain — provided a cause can be found — as well as develop a plan for treating the pain. However, you need to be careful. Not all doctors who claim to be pain specialists have received extensive training. Make sure you see a doctor who's certified in pain medicine.

Pain specialists

Pain specialists are doctors who work closely with your primary care physician to assess the cause of your pain and determine appropriate treatment. Doctors who have received extensive training in the treatment of pain often are board certified in the field of pain medicine. The types of doctors who most frequently specialize in pain management, and who are eligible for pain medicine certification, include the following:

- **Anesthesiologists.** These are doctors who are trained to relieve pain. In addition to preventing pain during and after surgery, anesthesiologists may also have specialty training in the treatment of chronic pain.

- **Neurologists.** Neurologists are doctors who diagnose and treat diseases of the nervous system.
- **Physiatrists.** Physiatrists are doctors who are trained in the field of physical medicine and rehabilitation, a branch of medicine that deals with treatment and prevention of disease by physical means, including exercise, manipulation and massage.
- **Psychiatrists.** Psychiatry is the branch of medicine devoted to the diagnosis and treatment of mental health disorders.

In addition to psychiatrists, some psychologists also specialize in the treatment of chronic pain. Because psychologists are not medical doctors, they aren't eligible for pain medicine certification. However, psychologists may receive accreditation from the American Board of Professional Psychology in Health.

Pain clinics

A pain clinic is the name often given to a medical facility that specializes in the treatment of chronic pain. Some facilities use the term *center* instead of *clinic*. A pain clinic, or center, may specialize in the treatment of a specific type of pain, such as headache or back pain, or it may treat an array of painful conditions.

Some pain clinics are associated with a medical institution, such as a pain clinic located within a hospital or medical center. Other pain clinics are stand-alone facilities that are run by one or more individual doctors.

Another way in which pain clinics differ is that some focus on only one type of pain treatment — for instance, the use of medication to relieve pain, either in the form of pills or injections. This compares with more broad-based pain clinics, which rely on a variety of treatments — from psychological counseling to physical therapy to acupuncture — to help manage pain.

Pain rehabilitation centers

With chronic pain, there often isn't an effective treatment that can make the pain go away. This can be a hard pill to swallow, especially if you've spent a lot of time and money hoping to relieve your pain. But it doesn't mean that all is lost. While you may not be able to make the pain disappear, you can learn how to cope with it.

With the right tools and techniques, it's possible to reduce your pain and improve your quality of life. Your doctor or a pain specialist may offer advice on how to manage your pain. You might also consider visiting a pain rehabilitation center, provided you live in a location with such a facility nearby, or you're willing to travel to a medical center that offers such a program. Pain rehabilitation programs are designed to reverse the downward course that can occur with chronic pain — helping you learn how to control your pain so that you can enjoy life, instead of letting your pain control you.

Rehabilitation programs

Pain rehabilitation programs support the belief that chronic pain affects many aspects of your life and, therefore,

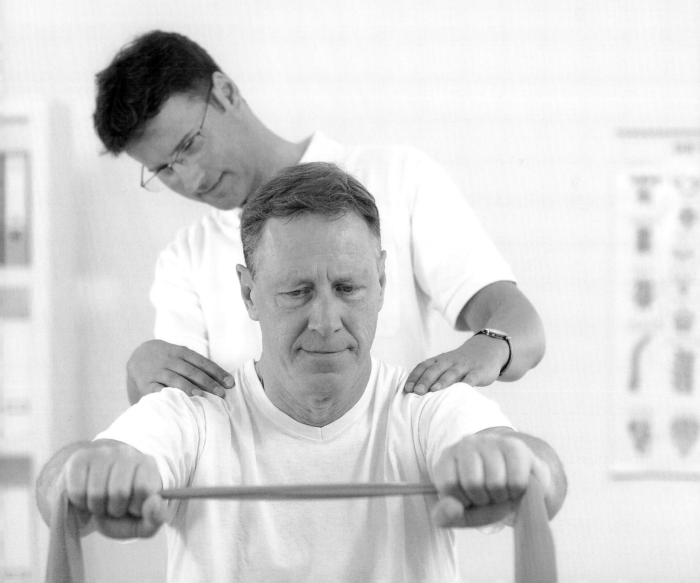

Is a pain rehabilitation program right for me?

Pain rehabilitation is a challenging process that requires a serious commitment. Ask yourself these questions to assess your readiness:

- Is my life controlled by pain?
- Are my doctors telling me they can do nothing further to relieve my pain?
- Am I concerned about the long-term effects of taking pain medications?
- Is my family's well-being affected by my pain?
- Is my recovery from injury or illness taking much longer than my doctors or I expected?
- Am I not able to commit to events with family or friends because of worry about controlling my pain?

requires a broad treatment approach. These programs explore various ways to help you control your pain. In addition, they help you identify factors that may contribute to your pain. The programs are generally intended for people who have experienced a significant decline in their daily functioning and quality of life as a result of their pain.

In most pain rehabilitation programs, pain specialists integrate behavioral and lifestyle changes with physical and occupational therapy and, occasionally, selective use of medications or injections. Depending on the location or cause of your pain, other therapies, such as relaxation techniques, stress management and complementary medicine, also may be incorporated into your treatment plan.

Most pain rehabilitation programs are located within large academic centers, and they include a large staff of doctors, nurses, psychologists, physical and occupational therapists, and other health professionals. The primary goal of these programs, which have been in existence for more than 30 years, is to restore physical functioning and improve the quality of life for people with unrelieved pain.

Goals of many programs include:

- Return to regular daily activities
- Elimination or reduction of pain medications that provide little or no benefit or cause adverse side effects
- Increased physical strength, stamina and flexibility
- Use of stress management and relaxation techniques
- Return to employment (if applicable)
- Resumption of leisure and recreational activities
- Improved relations with family, friends and co-workers
- Reduced reliance on health care professionals

What to expect

Not all pain clinics and rehabilitation programs operate exactly the same, but their approach is often quite similar. You'll likely receive a thorough evaluation. This may include having staff review your physical and psychological condition, use of medication, work situation, and relationships with family and friends. Additional diagnostic tests also may be performed.

Once the initial evaluation is complete, staff will work with you on different

ways to control the pain to keep it at a manageable level. They may also suggest that you set goals regarding what you hope to achieve during your time at the clinic or rehabilitation center. Your goals might include getting off your medication, becoming more physically active, learning to relax or returning to work.

With some rehabilitation programs, the therapy and attention you receive are intensive. You spend most of the day at the center for two to four weeks. During this time, you work with physical and occupational therapists and spend time in group sessions. You also meet regularly with your case manager to discuss your progress, as well as areas that remain difficult for you. With other rehabilitation programs, the schedule is less intensive. You meet for just a few hours a week over several weeks.

Working as a team

Doctors who specialize in the treatment of chronic pain often don't work alone. This is especially true for broad-based pain clinics and programs that treat a variety of conditions and that

Are pain rehabilitation programs effective?

Mayo Clinic's Comprehensive Pain Rehabilitation Center, founded in 1974, was one of the first pain rehabilitation centers in the United States. It's now one of the largest in the nation. The center offers an intensive three-week program that serves approximately 400 people annually.

As part of its mission to help people with chronic pain improve their quality of life, the center conducts ongoing research as to the effectiveness of the program. Treatment outcomes from individuals who have completed Mayo's program, shown below, are likely comparable to those at other reputable pain rehabilitation centers across the country. Participants were able to retain these benefits for at least six months.

Patient satisfaction

The majority of participants — 91 percent — "strongly agreed" or "agreed" that the pain rehabilitation center was beneficial in helping them learn how to live well in spite of chronic pain.

Medication

Upon completion of the program, 4 percent of participants were still taking opioid (narcotic) medications, compared with 45 percent at admission. Use of nonsteroidal anti-inflammatory drugs (NSAIDs) and muscle relaxants also decreased.

Depression

Scores on the Center for Epidemiological Studies Depression Scale showed a 79 percent reduction from admission to discharge among people experiencing depressive symptoms.

Physical therapy

Seventy-five percent of people completing the program had at least a 50 percent gain in their aerobic activity level. More than 20 percent of participants experienced a gain of 75 percent or more in their level of aerobic activity.

Pain severity

In rehabilitation, pain reduction is not a program goal, and there are no medical or surgical procedures to specifically reduce pain. However, because participants learn coping strategies for managing pain while improving the quality of their life, 73 percent of those completing the program report a reduction in the severity of their pain.

Confidence level

Eighty-four percent of participants note increased feelings of control over pain and life events.

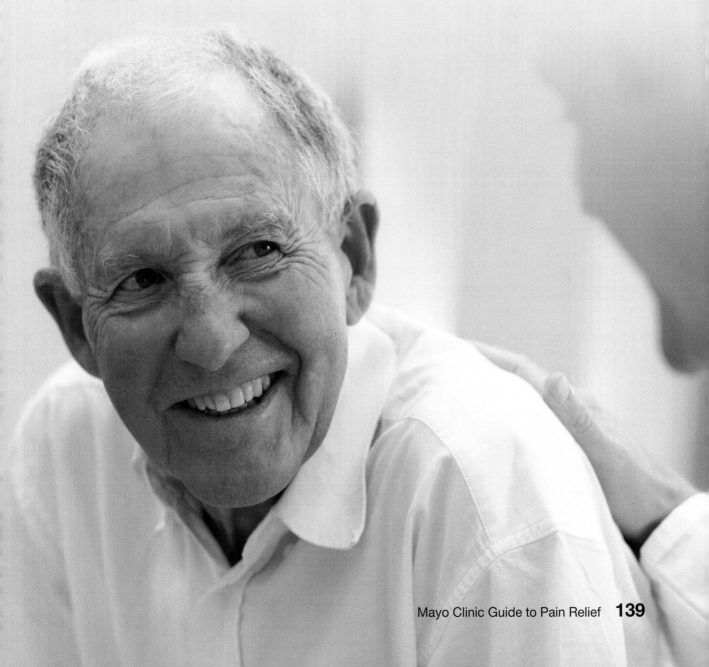

use a multifaceted approach to managing pain. In this type of setting, a pain specialist may lead or be part of a team that may include some or all of the following medical professionals:

Other doctors

In addition to specialists in pain medicine, the facility may also include other doctors who treat specific forms of pain, including anesthesiologists, neurologists, psychiatrists, or physical medicine and rehabilitation physicians (physiatrists).

Psychologists

Psychologists teach strategies to cope with pain and improve daily functioning. They also address behavioral and emotional issues that can accompany chronic pain, such as depression and fear, and they identify issues that may be contributing to the pain, such as strained family relations or stress.

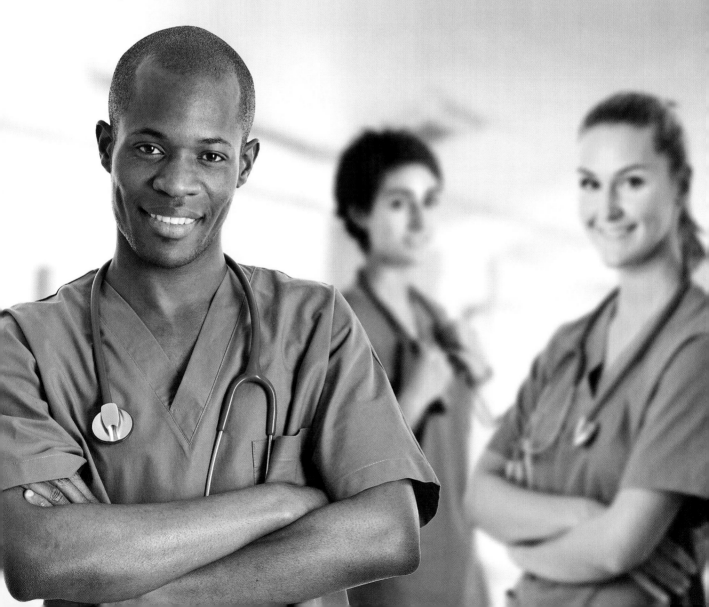

Nurses

Nurses often oversee medication use or medication withdrawal. They may monitor your progress and act as a case manager, serving as your advocate and acting as an intermediary to other professionals on the team.

Physical and occupational therapists

The role of therapists is to help rebuild your strength and endurance and to instill confidence in your ability to function in daily life. Physical therapists do this through individualized instruction in a complete exercise and fitness program. Occupational therapists, meanwhile, focus on increasing your competency in specific day-to-day tasks.

Others

Additional professionals may include a registered dietitian, a social worker and a vocational counselor.

What to look for

To find a reputable pain program that fits your needs, talk with your doctor. Organizations that may provide references include the American Pain Society and the American Academy of Pain Medicine (see page 266). Because pain clinics and programs vary in their qualifications and specialties, consider these factors when evaluating your options:

- **What are the goals of the program?** Is the program focused strictly on relieving your pain with specific interventions or medications? Or does it include a spectrum of services to help determine the cause of your pain or personal problems that may be associated with your pain?
- **What methods does the program advocate?** Be cautious of programs that advocate long-term use of potentially addictive drugs, such as narcotics, or that routinely include surgery or rely on unproven alternative therapies.
- **Are staff members friendly and willing to listen?** It's important that you feel comfortable with those around you. Staff should be interested in you and willing to take time to listen.
- **Is your doctor willing to answer questions?** Questions may include Do you have experience in treating my kind of pain? How long have you been practicing? Are you certified in pain management?
- **Is the program accredited or certified?** Pain centers or clinics don't have to be accredited or certified to operate. However, certification

helps ensure the program meets basic requirements.

- **Does it have a good success rate?** Ask what the long-term success rate of the program is. Keep in mind that no clinic or center can offer a 100 percent success rate.

- **Does it include follow-up services?** If you need additional care once you've completed your treatment, there should be a phone number to call or person to contact.

- **How much does it cost?** Know approximately what the treatment will cost before you start. Check with your insurance company to see what expenses are covered. Some insurance companies cover treatment provided by pain programs, while others don't.

- **What can I expect from participation in the program?** If providers promise complete relief of pain, this may not be realistic. Learning how to function in daily life despite some ongoing pain is a more realistic goal.

Chapter 10

Complementary and alternative medicine

In your quest to find relief from your pain, chances are you've tried or considered some form of complementary or alternative medicine. Maybe you've had a massage, practiced meditation or yoga, or thought about acupuncture.

And you probably have a lot of questions. Do these methods really work? Are they safe? Exactly what is complementary and alternative medicine? This chapter helps answer these questions.

The National Center for Complementary and Alternative Medicine (NCCAM), a division of the National Institutes of Health, defines complementary and alternative medicine as a group of diverse medical and health care practices and products that are generally not considered part of conventional medicine.

Complementary medicine refers to therapies used in addition to conventional treatments. An example would be practicing meditation in addition to taking prescription drugs to manage anxiety. In contrast, alternative medicine includes treatments used in place of traditional medicine. This might include seeing a homeopath or naturopath instead of your regular doctor.

Among the general public, however, this distinction isn't as clear. Many people use the term *alternative medicine* as a catchall phrase to refer to both — those therapies used in addition to conventional care and those used in place of it.

Integrative medicine, meanwhile, is a fairly new term that describes a growing movement taking place in many health care institutions — integrating complementary and alternative therapies with conventional medicine. The goal of integrative medicine is to treat the whole person — mind, body and spirit — not just the disease. This is done by combining the best of today's high-tech medicine with the best of nontraditional practices — treatments that have some high-quality evidence to support their use.

Complementary and alternative therapies aren't new. Some have been practiced for thousands of years. But their use has become more popular as people seek greater control of their own health.

Two of the most common conditions for which people use complementary and alternative medicine are anxiety and pain. Studies sponsored by NCCAM have shown that certain therapies, such as acupuncture, biofeedback, meditation and relaxed breathing, can be useful in treating chronic pain. For others, the evidence isn't as supportive.

5 smart strategies

Complementary and alternative medicine can play a role in better health. But it's important to remember that

there are some important differences between conventional medicine and complementary and alternative therapies and practices.

If you decide to use complementary and alternative treatments, protecting your health — and your wallet — requires you to do two things. First, find out how various treatments work and what benefits they may provide. Second, take responsibility for your own well-being. Before selecting a specific treatment, do your homework.

1. **Gather information about the treatment.** The Internet is one way to keep up with the latest on complementary and alternative treatments — a fast-changing field. But keep in mind that not everything posted on the Internet is true or reliable. In addition to the information you gather on the Internet, check with other sources, including people who've received the treatment.
2. **Find and evaluate treatment providers.** Don't be afraid to talk with your doctor. He or she may be familiar with practitioners in the area and be able to guide you to reliable providers. Whenever possible, talk to people who've been to the provider you're considering.

Too good to be true?

The Food and Drug Administration and the National Council Against Health Fraud recommend that you watch for the following claims or practices to protect yourself against potentially fraudulent treatments:

- Promotional materials include words such as *breakthrough*, *magical* or *new discovery*. If the product were in fact a cure, it would be widely reported in the media and your doctor would prescribe it.
- Promotional materials include pseudomedical jargon such as *detoxify*, *purify* or *energize*. Such claims are difficult to measure.
- The manufacturer claims that the product can treat a wide range of diseases and conditions. No single product can do this.
- The product is supposedly backed by scientific studies, but references aren't provided, are limited or are out-of-date.
- The product's promotional materials mention no negative side effects, only benefits.
- The manufacturer accuses the government or medical profession of suppressing important information about the product's benefits.

Before you receive a treatment, schedule an informational appointment to learn more about the procedure or therapy. With any treatment that you consider, determine if the benefits outweigh the risks.

3. **Consider treatment costs.** Many complementary and alternative approaches aren't covered by health insurance. Find out how much the treatment will cost you and get the total amount in writing before you start treatment.

4. **Check your attitude.** When it comes to complementary and alternative medicine, steer a middle course between uncritical acceptance and outright rejection. Learn to be open-minded and skeptical at the same time. Keep your mind open to different treatment options but evaluate them carefully.

5. **Opt for a combined approach.** Research indicates that the best use of unconventional medicine is to complement rather than replace

traditional medical care. Use complementary and alternative therapies in conjunction with the treatment being prescribed by your doctor.

While complementary and alternative therapies can help you maintain good health and relieve some symptoms, it's important that you continue to rely on conventional medicine to diagnose a problem and treat your condition. Make sure to tell your health care team about all of the treatments you're using — both conventional and unconventional.

Remember that there's no substitute for a healthy lifestyle. Nutrition, exercise, stress management and adequate rest are key to better health and pain relief.

Herbs and other supplements

As anyone who's walked through a health food store can attest, the profusion of herbal remedies and other dietary supplements is almost overwhelming. Following are some products heavily marketed for pain relief — especially arthritic pain.

Devil's claw

The herb devil's claw originates from the Kalahari desert region of southern Africa. It's used to relieve pain and inflammation in joints and to treat headache and back pain. The manner in which it works is unknown. Research suggests devil's claw may be effective for short-term treatment of osteoarthritic pain, and it may also help alleviate low back pain. But the studies have been small, and more information is needed before any recommendations can be made regarding its use.

Glucosamine and chondroitin

Glucosamine and chondroitin are natural compounds found in cartilage — the tough tissue that cushions joints. They're used to treat osteoarthritis, a painful condition caused by the inflammation, breakdown and loss of cartilage. Glucosamine supplements are made from the skeletons of shellfish (chitin). Chondroitin supplements are made from shark, cow or plant products, as well as from other sources.

Glucosamine and chondroitin have become an extremely popular treatment

Evaluating herbal remedies

Unlike medications you receive from your doctor, dietary and herbal products aren't regulated by the Food and Drug Administration for effectiveness. Regulations regarding the safety of these products also are different.

With prescription drugs, the manufacturer must prove that the benefits of the drug outweigh any safety concerns before the drug is approved for sale. Dietary and herbal supplements, however, are assumed to be safe until proved otherwise. Only when a supplement is found unsafe is it removed from the market. Because these products don't follow the same safety procedures, they can contain toxic substances that may not be listed on the label. In addition, the amount of active ingredient may vary greatly between different brands.

You might consider herbal products to be natural and, therefore, harmless. However, they can have active chemicals that may not safely mix with other medications you're taking. The best advice is to talk with your doctor before taking any dietary supplement or herbal product.

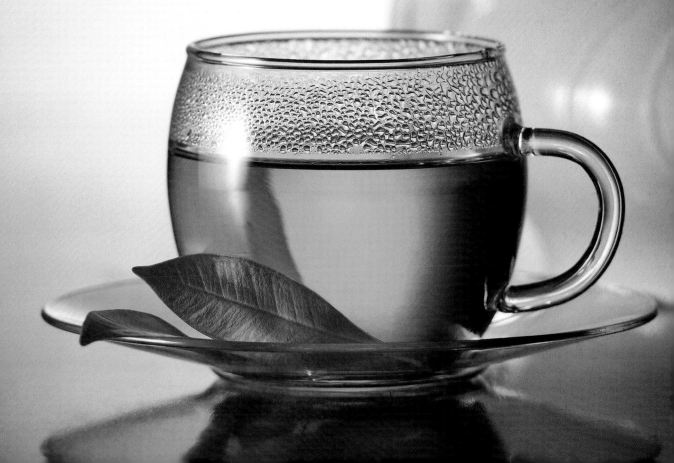

for osteoarthritis. They appear to be safe and produce fewer adverse side effects than do medications such as nonsteroidal anti-inflammatory drugs (NSAIDs). The question is, are they effective at treating arthritis?

While many older studies gave very promising results, the results of a large study sponsored by the National Institutes of Health (NIH) raised some questions. In that study, only individuals with very severe symptoms appeared to receive some benefit. The NIH study, however, was faced with a lot of challenges, and many questions still remain. But while the studies may be conflicting, side effects from the supplements are few and far between.

So far, no other treatments have shown promise at increasing cartilage. It's possible — though certainly not guaranteed — glucosamine and chondroitin may help.

SAMe

S-adenosyl-L-methionine (SAMe) is a compound that occurs naturally in the human body. Among other functions, it helps produce and regulate hormones and maintain cell membranes. Trials indicate that SAMe can relieve pain from osteoarthritis as effectively as NSAIDs, with fewer side effects.

But the long-term benefits and risks of SAMe are still unknown. As with any supplement, it's best to consult your doctor before trying SAMe. One drawback of SAMe is that it can interact with antidepressant medications. That is why, with any supplement that you take, it is important to talk with your doctor first.

Hands-on therapies

This group includes some of the most commonly used complementary treatments. Hands-on therapies are used to treat musculoskeletal conditions such as back pain, headache and arthritis.

Aromatherapy

This ancient form of healing involves the use of essential oils that are derived from plant extracts and resins and used to induce relaxation and promote both health and healing. Practitioners believe these oils can help treat various symptoms and conditions — including pain — when massaged into your skin or inhaled.

There are about 150 different essential oils used in aromatherapy. The oils are categorized according to their effects on the mind and body and on specific diseases. More study is needed to determine whether these oils provide any health benefit, and for which conditions they may be the most beneficial. Aromatherapy is often used in conjunction with massage therapy.

Chiropractic

Chiropractic therapy is perhaps the most common complementary therapy in the United States. It's based on the concept that restricted movement in the spine may lead to pain and reduced function. Spinal adjustment (manipulation) is one form of therapy chiropractors use to treat restricted spinal mobility. The goal is to restore spinal movement and, as a result, improve function and decrease back pain.

Studies have found spinal manipulation to be an effective treatment for uncomplicated low back pain, especially if the pain has been present less than four weeks. Studies also suggest spinal manipulation may be effective for headache and other spine-related conditions, such as neck pain. There's no evidence, though, to support the belief that spinal manipulation can cure whatever ails you.

As with any medical specialist, select a chiropractor who's willing to work with the other members of your health care team. Make sure you're comfortable with the recommendations, including how many sessions you'll need. Be questionable of chiropractors who ask to extend your treatment indefinitely.

When limited to the low back, chiropractic treatment has few risks. However, manipulation of the neck has been associated with injury to blood vessels supplying the brain. Rarely, neck manipulation may cause a stroke.

Massage

Massage therapy involves the use of different manipulative techniques to move your body's muscles and soft tissues. Massage therapists primarily use their hands to manipulate muscles and tissues, but sometimes they may use their forearms, elbows or feet.

There are many theories as to how massage therapy promotes good health.

One popular theory follows the belief that when muscles are overworked, waste products can accumulate in the muscle, causing soreness and stiffness. The aim of massage therapy is to improve circulation in the muscle, increasing the flow of nutrients and oxygen and eliminating waste products. Massage therapy also induces the body's relaxation response, another route to healing and improved health.

Massage therapists claim the treatment can help relieve stress and anxiety, relax your muscles, reduce headaches, lower blood pressure, improve range of motion in your joints, and increase the body's production of natural painkillers.

A growing body of literature is beginning to validate many of the benefits of massage therapy. Studies suggest it can decrease headache pain and pain associated with fibromyalgia. It may also help relieve back pain. Although massage is generally safe, avoid it if you have open sores, acute inflammation or circulatory problems. A massage should feel good. If it doesn't, speak up.

Movement therapies

Several nontraditional therapies, such as the Feldenkrais and Trager methods, center around the philosophy that, over time, people start moving and hold-

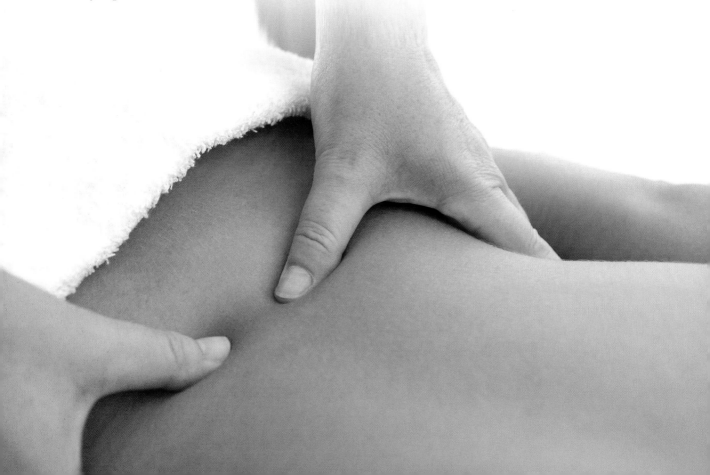

ing their bodies in dysfunctional ways. Weaker muscles end up doing the work of stronger muscles, causing stress and tension.

With these therapies, an instructor takes you through a series of specific movements designed to teach you to use your muscles and joints more comfortably and efficiently. The movements are also designed to help you find greater ease with your body.

Practitioners claim these therapies can help control pain and promote an overall sense of well-being. Although they appear to be safe, studies documenting their benefits are fairly limited.

Prolotherapy

Prolotherapy — also known as sclerotherapy or proliferant therapy — is a procedure done by a trained professional that involves injecting sterile solutions containing dextrose, a specific type of sugar, into painful ligaments and tendons. The solutions are intended to stimulate the production of connective tissue.

Proponents of prolotherapy believe the treatments help restore strength and stability to ligaments and joints, which

in turn helps relieve pain. Prolotherapy has been used to treat a number of painful musculoskeletal conditions, such as osteoarthritis and chronic back pain.

Studies of prolotherapy have produced conflicting evidence regarding its effectiveness in treating chronic pain. Some have suggested a possible benefit, while others have indicated none. At this point, more research is needed to determine what role, if any, prolotherapy may play in the treatment of chronic pain.

Rolfing

Rolfing is a form of deep-tissue massage. It's based on the theory that tissues surrounding your muscles become thickened and stiff as you get older. This affects your posture and how well you're able to move. The purpose of Rolfing is to align your body so that all of its components are positioned correctly.

Practitioners of Rolfing believe that injury or stress causes tissues to adhere in unhealthy ways, interfering with your body's natural movement and producing symptoms such as pain. To restore natural alignment, deep pressure is applied to stretch the tissues and help reposition muscles and joints.

Few scientific studies support Rolfing's benefits. Its deep massage may help reduce stress and tension. However, some people find the procedure painful, and it may worsen your pain.

Energy therapies

Energy therapies are based on the belief that the body contains natural energy fields and that good health results when this energy can flow freely without interruption.

Acupressure and acupuncture

These therapies stem from the Chinese belief that within the human body there are multiple invisible pathways, called meridians. Through these pathways flows qi (pronounced chee), the Chinese word for "life force" or "life energy." When the flow of qi is obstructed, illness or pain results.

During acupressure, a practitioner applies pressure with his or her fingers to specific points on your body in an attempt to restore the free flow of qi and relieve symptoms such as pain and stress. People who feel they're helped by the procedure find the therapy to be relaxing and comforting. However, more research is needed to document the effectiveness of this treatment.

During a typical acupuncture session, an acupuncturist inserts anywhere from one to 20 hair-thin needles into your skin for 10 to 30 minutes. The acupuncturist may also manipulate the needles or apply electrical stimulation or heat to the needles.

Acupuncture is one of the most studied nontraditional medical practices, and it continues to gain acceptance within modern medicine for treatment of certain conditions.

A number of studies have shown that acupuncture is effective in treating postoperative dental pain, pain related to endoscopic procedures, low back pain related to pregnancy and some forms of chronic pain, including fibromyalgic pain.

Acupuncture has also been effective in reducing pain related to tennis elbow, but it's had mixed results when used to treat osteoarthritis of the knee, hip and back. Some studies suggest it may provide considerable pain relief, while other studies show no benefit from the treatment.

Adverse side effects from acupuncture are rare, but they can occur. Make sure your acupuncturist is trained and certified or licensed and follows good hygiene practices, including use of disposable needles.

Magnet therapy

Most claims regarding the healing power of magnets are from manufacturers of products that contain magnets. These products include arm and leg wraps, belts, mattress pads and shoe inserts. Manufacturers often claim the products can relieve various health problems, including chronic pain, by stimulating your body's natural electrical field.

To date, there's no scientific evidence that magnets used in this manner provide any health benefits. And some experts believe inappropriate use of magnets could possibly lead to health problems.

A few medical researchers are exploring the use of different, more powerful magnets — not the common refrigerator magnets — as a therapy for some forms of chronic pain. More study is needed before any conclusions can be drawn.

Mind-body therapies

A simple definition of mind-body medicine reads like this: "positively influencing the mind to improve the health of the individual." The belief that mind and body are intricately connected goes back centuries. Mind-body practices have two core components. The first is to restore the mind to a state of peaceful neutrality. The second is to use this "ready" mind to improve your health.

Biofeedback

Biofeedback uses technology to teach you how to develop certain body responses that may help reduce your pain. During a biofeedback session, a trained therapist applies electrodes and other sensors to various parts of your body. The electrodes are attached to devices that monitor and give you feedback on body functions, including muscle tension, brain wave activity, respiration, heart rate, blood pressure and temperature.

Once the electrodes are in place, the therapist uses relaxation techniques to calm you, reducing muscle tension and slowing your heart rate and breathing.

You then learn how to produce these changes yourself. The goal of biofeedback is to help you enter a relaxed state in which you can better cope with your pain. Sometimes, specific muscle groups are monitored to help you learn how to position yourself in order to reduce muscle strain.

Biofeedback is, for the most part, widely used and accepted. It has the potential to improve symptoms associated with many medical conditions. It has relatively few risks, and it's practiced in many medical centers.

Studies indicate biofeedback has the potential to improve symptoms of headache, anxiety, stress, irritable bowel syndrome and high blood pressure, in addition to improving symptoms of other conditions, such as asthma, nausea and vomiting associated with chemotherapy and incontinence. Research is ongoing.

Hypnosis

People have been using hypnosis to promote healing since ancient times. Hypnosis produces an induced state of relaxation in which your mind stays narrowly focused and open to suggestion. It's not known how hypnosis works, but experts believe it alters your brain wave patterns in much the same way as other relaxation techniques.

For treatment of chronic pain, you receive suggestions designed to help you decrease your perception of the pain and increase your ability to cope with it. Unlike situations sometimes portrayed in movies and on TV, you can't be forced under hypnosis to do something you normally wouldn't want to do.

The success of hypnosis depends on your understanding of the procedure and your willingness to try it. You need to be strongly motivated to change. About 80 percent of adults can be hypnotized by a trained professional. People who don't want to feel out of control often can't be hypnotized.

The National Institutes of Health cites evidence that supports the effectiveness of hypnotherapy in the treatment of chronic pain associated with cancer, irritable bowel syndrome, temporal mandibular joint (TMJ) problems and some types of headache. Studies also show that hypnosis may reduce anxiety. Particularly, hypnosis has been shown to lower anxiety before some medical and dental procedures.

Meditation

The term *meditation* refers to a group of techniques, many of which have their roots in religious or spiritual traditions. Today, many people use meditation for health and wellness purposes.

In meditation, a person focuses attention on his or her breathing or on repeating a word, phrase or sound in order to suspend the stream of thoughts that normally occupies the conscious mind. Meditation is believed to lead to a state of physical relaxation, mental calmness, alertness and psychological balance. Practicing meditation can change how you respond to your brain's constant flow of emotions and thoughts, and it may help control how you react to a challenging situation.

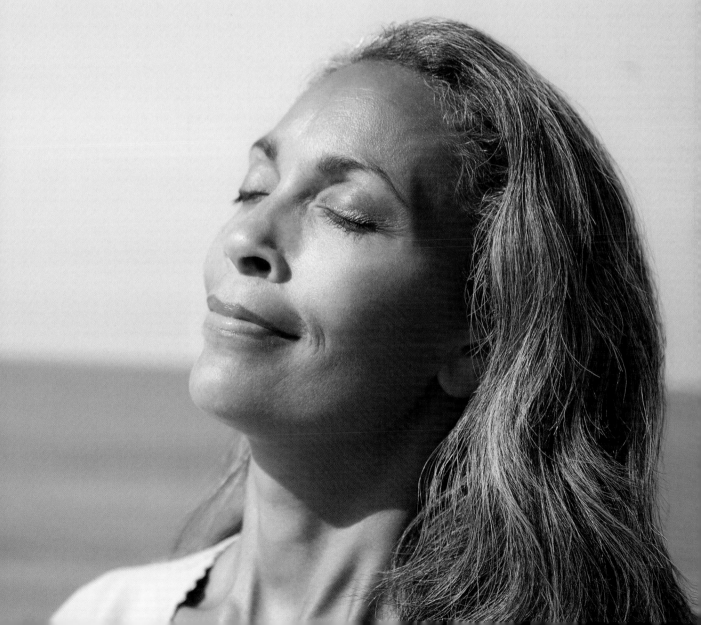

Meditation may be practiced on its own or as a part of another mind-body therapy, such as yoga or tai chi. Like these other therapies, once you learn how, you can meditate by yourself.

Meditation may be used to treat a number of problems, including anxiety, pain, depression, stress and insomnia. It can be the perfect complement to the rush of a busy, complicated life. As evidence supporting the use of meditation grows, adding it to your daily schedule may be just the antidote you need to deal with a hectic routine. In addition, if meditation helps lower your blood pressure and reduce stress, so much the better. The long-term benefits of meditation continue to be studied.

Music therapy

Practitioners of music therapy claim that it can lower stress, reduce symptoms of depression and promote pain relief. With this treatment, a trained music therapist uses music and all of its facets — physical, emotional, mental, social and spiritual — to help individuals improve or maintain their health. Performing or listening to music, with guidance from a music therapist, can help relieve muscle tension and slow your breathing.

Music therapy hasn't been extensively researched. However, it poses virtually no risk and is an inexpensive form of therapy. Several organizations promote the use of music for health and healing.

Tai chi

Tai chi, a form of martial arts developed in China, is a popular method for strengthening muscles, improving joint flexibility and reducing stress.

Tai chi involves gentle, deliberate circular movements, combined with deep breathing. As you concentrate on the motions of your body, you develop a feeling of tranquility. For this reason, tai chi is sometimes described as a form of moving meditation. Similar to other forms of Chinese medicine, it's designed to foster the free flow of qi necessary for health.

If you're trying to improve your general health, you may find tai chi helpful as part of your program. It is generally safe for people of all ages and levels of fitness. Studies show that for older adults it can improve balance and reduce the risk of falls.

Because the movements are low impact and they put minimal stress on your

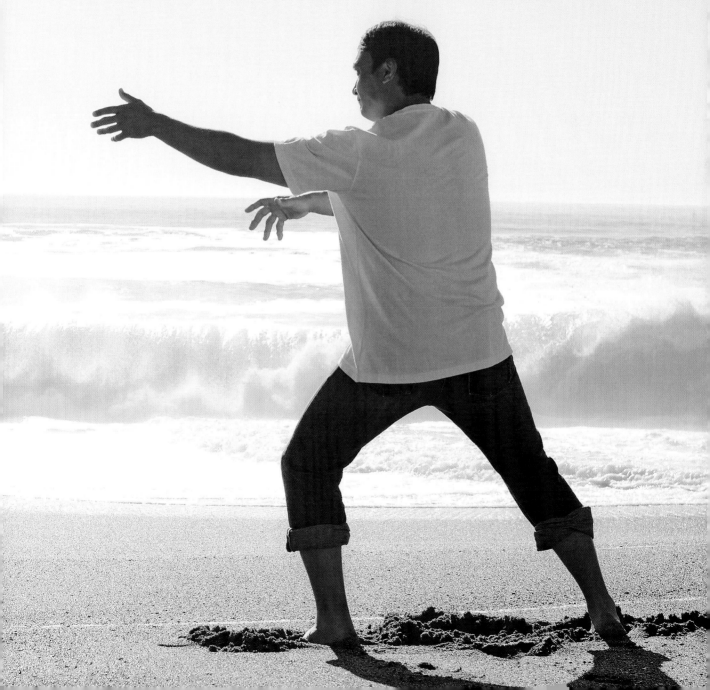

muscles and joints, tai chi is appealing to many. For these same reasons, if you have a condition such as arthritis or you're recovering from an injury, you may find tai chi useful. It may help you reduce your level of stress and manage conditions such as high blood pressure and depression.

Yoga

People practice yoga for many reasons. For some, it's a spiritual path. For others, it's a way to promote physical flexibility, strength and endurance. In either case, you may find that yoga can help you relax and manage stress.

The ultimate goal of yoga is to reach complete peacefulness of body and mind by way of breathing, meditation and posture. Traditional yoga philosophy also requires that practitioners adhere to ethical behavior and dietary practices. However, chances are you may not be looking for a complete change in lifestyle but rather a tool to help increase flexibility, promote relaxation or relieve stress.

According to the National Institutes of Health, yoga can help reduce stress, slow breathing, lower blood pressure and alter brain waves. Its precise, quiet movements focus your mind less on your busy day and more on the moment at hand, as you move your body through poses that require balance and concentration.

Part 3

Managing chronic pain

Chapter 11

Developing a pain control program

Many people with chronic pain enjoy active and productive lives. If you aren't among them, there's no reason you can't be. But it's up to you to make it happen.

In this chapter and those that follow, we discuss various steps you can take to help lessen your pain and make it more manageable. There aren't any quick fixes for chronic pain. And most often, you're the key ingredient. If you want your life to improve, you need to lead the way.

You may not like the fact that you have chronic pain. No one does. But clinging to unrealistic hopes or expectations will only prolong your frustration and contribute to your feelings of helplessness. The first and most important step in controlling chronic pain is accepting the fact that you may always have pain. While some people are able to significantly reduce or eliminate their pain, for many people it will always be a part of their lives. Managing chronic pain is about learning how to keep your pain at a tolerable level so that you can enjoy life.

The remainder of this book focuses on specific lifestyle issues and pain management strategies that can help you better understand and manage your pain. The task ahead may seem daunting, but each small step you take in your new role as pain manager will boost your self-confidence and strengthen your faith in your abilities.

The choice is yours to make. You can continue to dwell on your discomfort, or you can do something about it.

Start with SMART goals

Goal setting is an important part of your pain control program and your first step in achieving pain relief. Goals help divert your attention from your pain, and they provide an opportunity to think about your lifestyle and what you can do to better manage your pain. Goals also give you something to strive for.

But goal setting isn't as easy as it may sound. You simply can't identify some things that you want to occur and expect them to happen. You'll only be setting yourself up for disappointment.

In this chapter we talk about setting SMART goals — goals that are specific, measurable, attainable, realistic and timely. And in the remaining chapters, we give examples of how you can use the SMART formula in various aspects of your pain program.

Specific
Your goals should be clear and straightforward. State exactly what you want to achieve, how you're going to do it and when you want to achieve it. To begin with, set goals that you can achieve within a week to a month. It's easy to give up on goals that take too long to reach. You might even start off with a goal you can achieve the same day. If you have a big goal, break it down into a series of smaller weekly or daily goals. After you achieve one of the smaller goals, move on to the next.

Measurable
A goal doesn't do you any good if there's no way of telling whether you've achieved it. "I want to feel better" isn't a good goal because it's not specific and it's difficult to measure. "I want to be able to work eight hours a day" is a better goal because it's specific and measurable.

Attainable
Ask yourself whether the goal is within reasonable reach. Goals that are too far out of your reach you probably won't commit to doing. For instance, completing a marathon may not be an achievable goal if you've never run before. However, short hikes around the neighborhood or completing a 5K run may be attainable.

Realistic
Is the goal realistic for you? The purpose of a goal is to shift your focus from your pain to your future. But you can't ignore your limitations. Your goals need to be within your

How to be SMART

Here are examples of goals that follow the SMART formula:

Goal: Reduce my use of over-the-counter pain medications by 25 percent
When I want to achieve it: Two weeks
How I'm going to do it: Use other pain management strategies: exercise daily, pace myself at work and take frequent breaks, use relaxation techniques
How I'm going to measure it: Record in my journal daily the medication I took and how much

Goal: Exercise 20 minutes each day
When I want to achieve it: One week
How I'm going to do it: Stretch and do strengthening exercises five minutes in the morning, walk five minutes during my lunch hour, bicycle 10 minutes in the evening
How I'm going to measure it: Record in my journal when I exercised and for how long

capabilities. If you've suffered a serious back injury, a goal of returning to work as a bricklayer may not be realistic. Instead, your goal might be to find a sales job in a related field. Or you might decide to go back to school for training in a new field.

Timely

Set a time frame for your goal. When do you want to achieve it? Next week? In six months? Putting an end date on your goal gives you a clear target to work toward. If you don't set a comple-tion date, there's less reason to make a commitment.

What are your goals?

Think carefully about some short-term or long-term goals that you want to achieve. If you have some in mind, write them down now. Consider setting SMART goals for yourself in the following areas if you feel that they're aspects of your life that could use some improvement:

- Becoming more physically active
- Balancing work and leisure activities
- Managing your emotions and behaviors
- Reducing daily stress
- Enjoying time with family and friends
- Taking better care of your health
- Reducing use of medication (It's a good idea to discuss this with your doctor first.)

Put it in writing

As you begin to think about and set goals, something that you'll find helpful in tracking your progress is a daily journal (see "Sample journal" on page 166). In addition, a journal can help you determine those therapies or activities that seem to be helping you the most. As you work on your goals and you learn techniques to manage your pain, you should see a decrease in your pain level.

A journal can also open your eyes to aspects of your daily life that may be contributing to your pain. Many people think that their pain isn't influenced by factors such as work, stress, sleep or physical activity. But after a few months of tracking their pain levels and their activities, they begin to notice some common patterns. And they begin to see things in their lives that they can modify to improve their pain.

In addition, a journal can be a great way to express your feelings about your pain or other things that are happening in your life. Writing your thoughts and feelings on paper helps you organize and sort through problems and emotions and get them off your chest, similar to the way you feel after a good heart-to-heart visit with a friend or family member.

Here are things to consider keeping track of in your journal. You don't need to go into a lot of detail if you don't want to. Your journal can be as basic or as detailed as you want it to be.

Pain level and activities

In your journal, begin by recording your pain level. Health care professionals typically measure pain on a scale of 0 to 10, with 0 indicating no pain and 10 being the worst pain imaginable. Using this scale as your guide, rate your pain level and record it in your journal a couple of times a day.

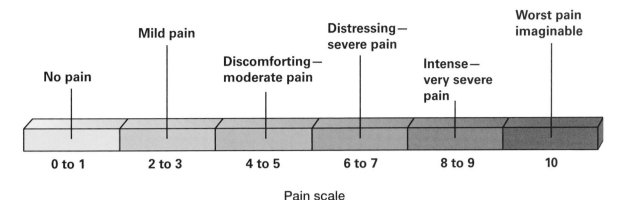

Pain scale

Use this scale as a guide when determining your level of pain.

You can do this whenever it's convenient, but keep the times consistent. Many people choose to record their pain level in the morning when they wake up, after lunch and then again in the evening before going to bed.

Keeping a log of your pain levels and activities allows you to:

Learn your pain pattern. Most people find the changes in their pain levels are quite consistent. For example, your pain may be at its lowest level in the morning and its highest level in the evening. Recording your pain levels helps you determine and analyze your pain pattern.

Link your pain with your activities. If your pain is the worst in the evening, why? Look to see if certain activities seem to correlate with an increase or a decrease in your pain level. Are you sitting or standing too long? Is your rush to get dinner ready a contributing factor? Are you just tired? Does isolation make your pain worse?

Identify flares. Recording your pain levels helps draw attention to inconsistencies. If your pain level at noon is normally a 3 and one day it's a 6, seeing the difference may prompt you to think about your morning. Did you do something different? You can also learn from days when your pain seems more tolerable. Was there something you did that may have lessened the pain?

See your progress. If you feel you aren't making progress, reading your journal may help you realize that your life has improved, even though the process may seem slow.

Sample journal

There is no right or wrong way when it comes to keeping a journal. Some people simply like to jot down their thoughts, and others prefer a worksheet format. This is just one example of how your journal might look and the information to include.

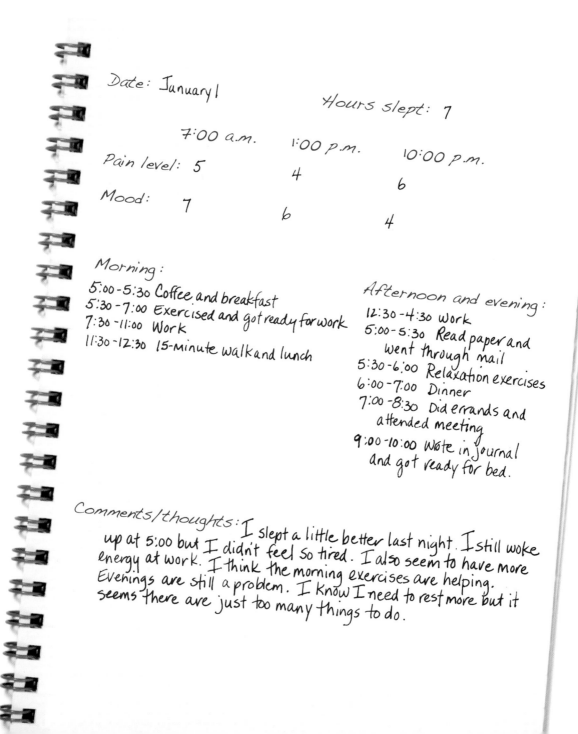

Date: January 1

Hours slept: 7

	7:00 a.m.	1:00 p.m.	10:00 p.m.
Pain level:	5	4	6
Mood:	7	6	4

Morning:
5:00-5:30 Coffee and breakfast
5:30-7:00 Exercised and got ready for work
7:30-11:00 Work
11:30-12:30 15-minute walk and lunch

Afternoon and evening:
12:30-4:30 Work
5:00-5:30 Read paper and went through mail
5:30-6:00 Relaxation exercises
6:00-7:00 Dinner
7:00-8:30 Did errands and attended meeting
9:00-10:00 Wrote in journal and got ready for bed.

Comments/thoughts: I slept a little better last night. I still woke up at 5:00 but I didn't feel so tired. I also seem to have more energy at work. I think the morning exercises are helping. Evenings are still a problem. I know I need to rest more but it seems there are just too many things to do.

Mood

On a scale of 0 to 10, with 0 being poor and 10 being excellent, rate your mood throughout the day. This exercise helps you realize that even though your pain and your mood are closely aligned, they aren't bound together.

Typically, the worse your pain, the worse your mood, and vice versa. As you begin to feel more in control of your pain, you may find your mood improving at a faster rate than the improvement in your pain levels. You begin to realize that even though you may not be able to eliminate your pain, you can learn to live with it and still be happy.

Sleep

A good night's sleep is important. It better equips you to handle your day. However, getting enough sleep can be difficult because your pain may keep you up at night. In contrast, some people spend too much time in bed. This can also reduce your tolerance to pain.

To help you get a better idea of how well you are — or aren't — sleeping, each day record how many hours you slept during the night and how many times you woke up. Eight hours is about average, but the amount of sleep each person needs varies. Your goal should be to feel rested when you wake up. If you're having trouble sleeping, tips to help you sleep better are discussed in Chapter 14.

Going forward

Up to this point, we've given you a lot of information regarding pain and various options for treating it. The chapters that follow are devoted to specific components of a pain management program. They include topics such as staying physically active, controlling your weight, reducing stress, finding a healthy balance of work and leisure activities, treating depression, and dealing with difficult emotions and behaviors.

In these chapters, you'll learn about specific steps that you can take to help manage your pain and improve your daily functioning. As you read through these chapters, keep in mind how the two key components outlined here — goal setting and daily journaling — can help you be successful in your efforts to enjoy life with less pain.

Finding the right doctor

Taking charge of your pain doesn't mean that you shouldn't seek help from others. Having people who can help you when you have questions or you need assistance is important. A doctor can be especially helpful. But make sure it's a doctor who understands your condition and believes in what you're doing.

The right doctor for you could be your family physician or a specialist who's overseeing your condition. Or you may want to see a doctor or a psychologist who specializes in pain management (see Chapter 9). If you're not sure where to find a pain specialist, ask your primary care doctor to refer you to one. Before selecting a new doctor, however, check with your health insurance provider to make sure that the care will be covered under your policy.

When selecting a doctor, look for someone who:

- Is knowledgeable about chronic pain
- Wants to help
- Listens well
- Makes you feel at ease
- Encourages you to ask questions
- Seems honest and trustworthy
- Allows you to disagree
- Is willing to talk with your family or friends

In addition to finding the right doctor, make an effort to learn all that you can about your condition and your pain. This will make it easier for the two of you to work together as a team.

Chapter 12

Staying active with daily exercise

There was a time when people with chronic pain were told to avoid physical activity for fear it would damage their joints and muscles and worsen their pain.

A common misconception is that exercise aggravates pain. To the contrary, exercise can help reduce it. During physical activity, your body releases chemicals called endorphins and enkephalins that block pain signals from reaching your brain. These chemicals also help alleviate anxiety and depression, conditions that can make your pain more difficult to control. Exercise also strengthens muscles and ligaments, reducing stress on painful joints.

However, many people bothered by chronic pain don't exercise. Perhaps you're one of them. Maybe you tried exercising, but when you did so the next day your pain was worse so you quit. This is commonly referred to as the "crash and burn" experience. When you first begin to exercise, your pain may worsen before it improves. The key is to increase your activity level gradually. It's also important to make exercise a daily habit. With time, you'll have less pain and you'll feel better about yourself.

The pages that follow contain information about specific types of exercise that can help improve your activity level and, in turn, reduce your pain. The exercises fall into three categories:

- Exercises to improve flexibility
- Exercises to improve aerobic capacity
- Exercises to build strength

Before you get started

It's always a good idea to talk with your doctor before starting any type of physical activity program. If you have another health problem or you're at risk of cardiovascular disease, you may need to take some precautions while you exercise.

It's especially important that you see your doctor if you:

- Have a blood pressure of 160/100 millimeters of mercury or higher
- Have diabetes or heart, lung or kidney disease
- Are a man age 40 or older or a women age 50 or older and haven't had a recent physical examination
- Have a family history of heart-related problems before age 55
- Are unsure of your health status
- Have previously experienced chest discomfort, shortness of breath or dizziness during exercise or strenuous activity

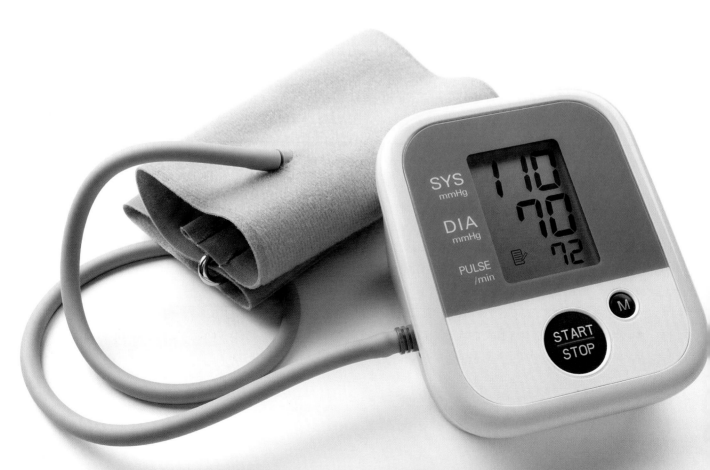

Flexibility exercises

Flexibility exercises include range-of-motion and stretching exercises. They help ease movement in your joints, allowing you to carry out daily activities more comfortably. They also help prevent your muscles from shortening and tightening, which can increase your risk of injury.

Range-of-motion exercises

Include some or all of the exercises on the following pages in your physical activity program. With each exercise, move slowly and easily. Repeat each exercise five times, and then move on to the next.

Neck
- Bring your chin toward your chest. Then return to normal position. Avoid extending your neck too far back, as this can worsen neck pain.
- Tilt your left ear toward your left shoulder. Return to normal position and tilt your right ear toward your right shoulder. Return to normal position. Avoid raising your shoulder toward your head.
- Turn your face to the left, then to the right. Keep your neck, shoulders and trunk straight.

Jaw
- Open your mouth as wide as possible without clicking or popping. Then close your mouth.
- Move your jaw to the right, then to the left.
- Move your jaw forward, then back.

Shoulders
- Put your arms at your sides.
- Roll your shoulders forward in a circular motion. Reverse.
- Bring your arms forward and over your head. Keep your trunk straight.
- Raise your arms from your sides to over your head. Keep your trunk straight and your palms up.

- Bring your elbows to shoulder height. Pull your elbows backward and feel a stretch in your chest muscles.

Elbows
- Bend and straighten your elbows.
- Keeping your arms next to your body, bend your elbows to make a right angle and turn your palms up and down.

Wrists
- Move your hands from side to side as far as possible, bending at the wrists in a fanning motion.
- Move your hands up and down, bending at the wrists and using a chopping motion.

Fingers and thumbs
- Bend your fingers to make a fist. Then fully straighten them.
- Bend your fingers at the knuckles, forming a claw. Then straighten them.
- Bend your thumbs across your palms and pull toward your little fingers.
- Touch the tips of your thumbs to the tips of your little fingers. Open your hands wide. Repeat, touching your thumbs to each finger.

Hips
- March in place, bringing your knees up high.
- Raise your leg out to the side. Alternate legs.
- Lift your leg backward, keeping your knee straight. Alternate legs.
- Kick your feet up behind you, by bending your knees.

Trunk
- Stand with your hands on your hips.
- Bend your upper body to the left. Repeat to the right.
- Twist your upper body to the right at your waist. Don't turn your pelvis. Repeat to the left.

Ankles and feet

- Stand with your feet about 12 inches apart.
- Rise on the toes of both feet. Relax to starting position. Rise on the toes of your right foot. Relax. Rise on the toes of both feet. Relax. Rise on the toes of your left foot. Relax.
- Walk on your heels.
- Walk on your toes.
- Walk heel to toe, as though you're on a tightrope.

Stretching exercises

Stretching each time you exercise helps to keep your muscles limber and to reduce tightness in the muscles.

Stretch slowly, holding the position for 30 to 60 seconds, and then slowly release. Breathe deeply and slowly while you stretch. Never bounce, and stretch only until you feel a noticeable pull. Your muscles respond to overstretching by tightening — the opposite of what you want.

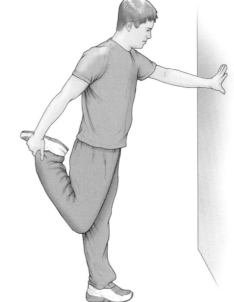

Quadriceps stretch

Stand facing a wall and place your left hand against the wall. Grasp the top of your right foot with your right hand and gently pull your foot or heel up toward your buttocks until you a feel mild tension in the front of your thigh. Hold your abdomen in and keep your back straight. Hold the stretch and repeat the movement with the other leg. This exercise may also be done while holding on to the back of a chair in front of you with both hands and pulling a foot up toward your buttocks (or as close as you can get) without holding on to the foot. Use the chair method if balancing on one foot is difficult.

Calf stretch

Stand at arm's length from a wall with your palms flat against the wall. Keep one leg back with your knee straight and your heel flat on the floor. Slowly bend your elbows and front knee and lean toward the wall until you feel a stretch of the back lower calf muscle. Hold. Repeat with the other leg.

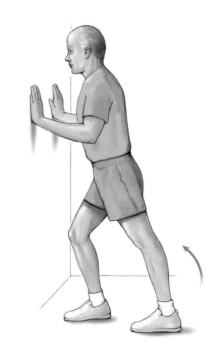

Gluteal stretch

Lie on the floor or a bed with both legs bent and your feet flat on the floor or bed. Pull your right thigh and knee firmly toward your chest until your lower back flattens against the floor or bed. Hold the stretch and repeat the movement with the other leg.

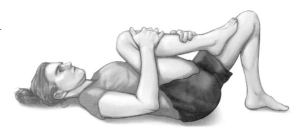

Lumbar stretch

Lie on the floor or a bed, with your knees bent. Pull both knees toward your chest until your lower back flattens against the floor or bed. Briefly hold the stretch and release. If knee pain is aggravated by this exercise, place your hands behind the knee joints when pulling your knees toward your chest. Avoid this exercise if you have osteoporosis or have undergone hip replacement.

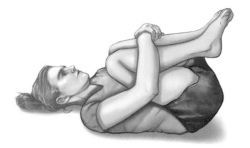

© MFMER

Hamstring stretch

Sit on a low chair with your leg propped on another chair in front of you. Without bending your knee, lean forward from your hips. Keep your back straight. Lean forward until you feel a gentle pull in the muscles under your thigh. Hold. Repeat with the other leg.

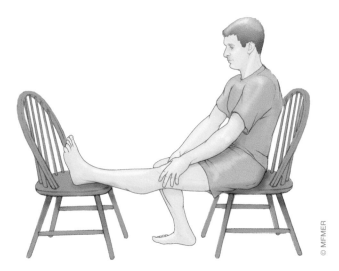

© MFMER

Looking for a helping hand?

For help with designing and getting started on an activity program, contact one of these professionals:

Physical therapist. A physical therapist is trained in the use of exercise to achieve physical fitness. He or she can help you select the most appropriate exercises based on the location of your pain and show you how to do the exercises properly. While a physical therapist can guide you, it's still up to you to do the exercises.

Occupational therapist. An occupational therapist can teach you how to perform daily activities — such as lifting, reaching and even getting dressed — in ways that won't place extra stress on your joints.

Certified exercise therapist. Many health clubs have employees who are trained in exercise therapy. If you belong to a health club — or are thinking of joining one — make an appointment to meet with a certified therapist for help with developing an exercise plan.

Aerobic exercises

Aerobic exercises place added demands on your heart, lungs and muscles, increasing your heart rate, blood pressure and need for oxygen. These exercises help your body work more efficiently and reduce your risk of cardiovascular disease, including heart attack and high blood pressure. Aerobic activity also increases your stamina, so you don't become easily fatigued and you have more energy for daily activities.

Aim for 20 to 30 minutes of moderately intense aerobic activity five days each week. If you've been inactive, you might start out by walking 10 minutes at a time, three times a day. Gradually increase your time and level of exertion until you are exercising five days a week.

There are many types of aerobic activity. Walking is the most common because it's easy to do, convenient and inexpensive. All you need is a good pair of walking shoes. Other aerobic exercises include:

- Aerobic dance
- Bicycling
- Cross-country skiing
- Dancing
- Golfing
- Hiking
- Swimming and water aerobics

What about weightlifting?

Lifting weights is an excellent way to strengthen your muscles. However, it's best to work with a physical therapist or fitness trainer in developing and beginning a weightlifting program. A therapist or trainer will help you select the appropriate weights for your level of fitness and teach you how to lift them properly to avoid injury to your muscles and joints.

Water aerobics has become increasingly popular among people with chronic pain because water's buoyancy reduces stress on your joints. Water also provides resistance to increase the benefits of aerobic activity. In addition, many people find warm water to be relaxing and soothing to sore muscles and joints.

A disadvantage of water exercises is that they aren't weight bearing. To maintain bone mass and protect against osteoporosis, combine water exercises with activities such as walking or lifting weights.

Strengthening exercises

Strong muscles improve your physical fitness and reduce fatigue. They also make it easier to carry out more vigorous types of daily activities, such as carrying laundry up and down stairs or lifting items at work.

To build muscle, include some or all of these exercises five days a week. If you're out of shape, begin with five repetitions of each and slowly build to 25 repetitions by adding one repetition each day.

Abdominal exercises

Lie on the floor or a firm surface with your knees bent. Raise your head and shoulders so that your shoulder blades lift off the floor or surface. Keep your head in a neutral position. Bring your head and shoulders back down. Don't do this exercise if you have osteoporosis.

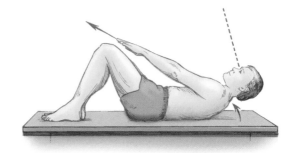

Repeat the stretch, reaching both hands toward your left knee. Relax and repeat with the right knee. Skip this exercise if it bothers your neck or you have osteoporosis.

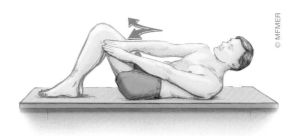

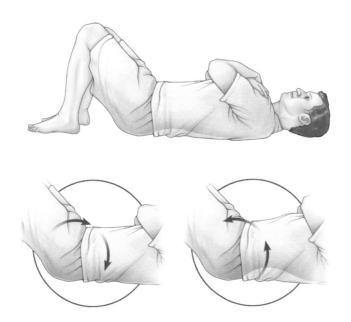

Lie on a firm surface with your knees bent. Place your hands across your chest. Tighten your stomach muscles, causing the small of your back to flatten against the surface. Hold for three to five seconds. Relax and repeat.

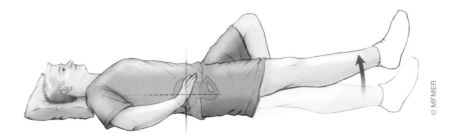

Lie on your back with your left knee bent and your right knee straight. Hold your abdominal muscles tight and slowly raise and lower your right leg. Relax and repeat. Reverse legs.

Back exercises

Sit upright in a chair (top). Put your hands on your hips or behind your back and squeeze your shoulder blades together. Hold for five seconds. Relax and repeat.

Lie facedown on top of one or two large pillows with a folded towel under your forehead (bottom). Position the pillow(s) under your bellybutton to keep your spine in a neutral position. Place your hands at your sides. Pulling your shoulder blades together, raise your head and chest. Keep your neck relaxed. Return to the starting position and repeat. Don't arch.

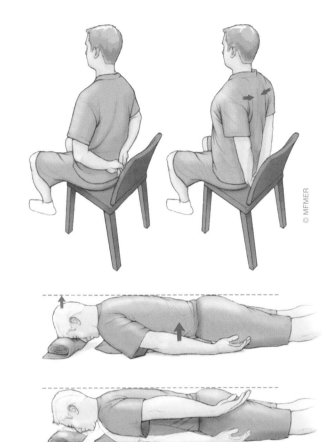

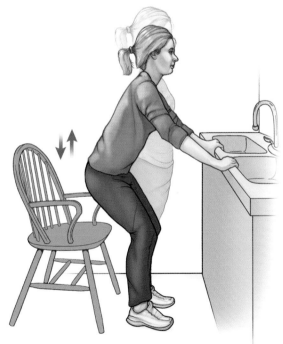

Leg exercises

Stand in front of a counter with a sturdy chair behind you. Hold on to the counter for support. Breathe out and squat down as far as you can comfortably go, keeping your knees in line with your toes. Hold the position for five seconds. Inhale and return to standing. Relax and repeat. As you build strength, hold the squat for longer or squat down farther.

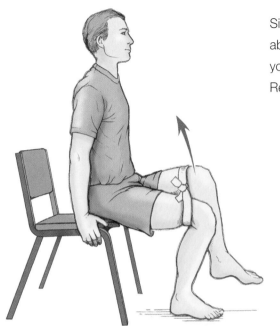

Sit on a chair. Weave a soft belt around your legs just above your knees so that it forms a figure eight. Pulling your legs in opposite directions, lift one leg off the floor. Relax. Repeat with other leg.

Sit on a chair or on a sturdy table. Weave a soft belt around your ankles so that it forms a figure eight. Try to straighten one leg while pulling the other foot backward, applying equal force with both legs. Gently push for three to five seconds. Relax. Repeat with the other leg.

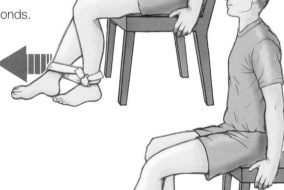

© MFMER

Perfecting your posture

Good posture places only minimal strain on your joints and muscles. Poor posture, however, can increase stress on some muscles, stretching them or causing them to shorten. When overstretched, your muscles lose their strength and are more prone to injury and pain.

Avoid poor posture. One extreme of poor posture when standing is the swayback. In this position, your stomach protrudes too far in front and your buttocks extend too far in the rear. This position puts excessive pressure on your lower back.

The opposite extreme is the slouch position, in which your shoulders are rolled forward. If you perpetually slouch, muscles in your chest shorten, reducing your flexibility.

Practice good posture. Good posture will help you relax your muscles and may reduce your pain. Throughout the day, including when you exercise, try to maintain good posture.

Standing posture
- Hold your chest high, keeping your shoulders back and relaxed.
- Gently pull your bellybutton toward your spine. Hold the position while breathing normally and looking straight ahead.
- Keep your feet parallel and your weight balanced on both feet.
- Keep your knees straight — not bent or in a locked position.

Sitting posture
- Rest both feel on the floor, keeping your knees level with your hips.
- Sit with your back pressed firmly against the chair. If necessary, support your lower back with a small cushion or rolled towel.
- Keep your upper back and neck comfortably straight, tucking your chin in slightly.
- Keep your shoulders relaxed — not elevated, rounded or pulled backward.

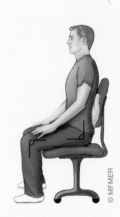

Chest and arm exercises

Sit in a sturdy chair that has arms. Keeping your spine straight, try raising yourself up off the chair without using your arms or hands to assist you. Relax and repeat. If your legs are weak or you have problems with balance, you may need to push your body up using your arms or hands. Skip this exercise if it causes pain to your hands, wrists or elbows.

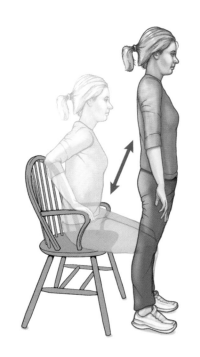

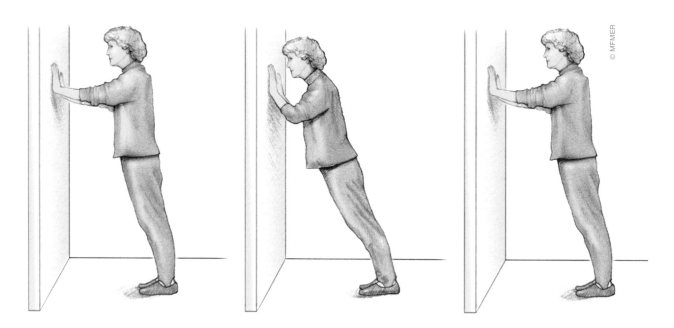

Stand facing a wall, far enough away that you can place your palms on the wall with your elbows slightly bent. Slowly bend your elbows and lean toward the wall. Straighten your arms and return to a standing position. Repeat. As you build strength, try standing farther from the wall.

This activity plan is safe for almost everyone. However, you still may want to discuss it with your doctor to make sure there aren't any exercises that you should avoid because of a physical condition or injury.

As you begin the program, remember to take it slow and gradually increase your level of activity. Don't try to do too much too soon. Flexibility, stretching and aerobic exercises can be done daily, or most days of the week. Include strengthening exercises at least three days a week. If your goal is to build strength in a weakened or painful joint, include strengthening exercises in your routine five days a week.

How to make it work

Regular exercise can help you stay active and allow you to continue to enjoy your favorite leisure activities. As

Get smart

Here are examples of exercise goals that follow the SMART formula:

Goal: Strengthen my knees to reduce the pain
When I want to achieve it: Three months
How I'm going to do it: Do strengthening exercises each morning; start with 15 minutes and build up to 30 minutes
How I'm going to measure it: Record in my journal each day when and for how long I exercised, and rate the level of pain in my knees

Goal: Have more energy
When I want to achieve it: Four weeks
How I'm going to do it: Walk for 15 minutes seven days a week and build up to 30 minutes daily
How I'm going to measure it: Record in my journal each day when and for how long I exercised

many people can attest, the difficulty with exercise is to keep it up — to make it a regular part of your daily routine.

You need to find ways to stay active and stay motivated. Here are some tips to get you started:

Set some goals

Start with simple goals and then progress to longer range goals. People who can stay physically active for six months usually end up making regular activity a habit. Remember to make your goals realistic and attainable (see page 162). It's easy to get frustrated and give up on goals that are too ambitious.

Have a game plan

Decide what time of the day you're going to exercise, what exercises you're going to do — flexibility, aerobic or strength — and for how long you are going to do them. You don't have to do them all at once. For instance, you might do 15 minutes of flexibility exercises in the morning, take a short break and then walk for 20 minutes. In the afternoon, make time for 15 minutes of strengthening exercises.

Don't be a weekend warrior

The most common mistakes people make are starting an exercise program at too high an intensity and progressing too quickly. The resulting pain and stiffness the next day can be very discouraging. It's better to progress slowly and stay within your capacity.

Shake it up

Vary what you do to prevent boredom. For example, try alternating walking and bicycling with swimming or a low-impact aerobic dance class. On days when the weather is pleasant, do your flexibility or stretching exercises outside.

Put it in writing

To begin with, record what you do each time you exercise, how long you do it, and how you feel during and after exercising. Logging your efforts helps you work toward your goals and reminds you that you're making progress.

Give yourself a pat on the back

After each exercise session, take two to five minutes to relax. Think about what you've just accomplished. This type of internal reward can help you make a long-term commitment to regular exercise.

Chapter 13

Balance, moderation and changing habits

How you organize and go about your day can significantly affect your ability to manage your pain. If you overdo it to meet a deadline at work or you overcommit yourself so that you're running from one activity to the next, your body reaches a point where it can't keep up. Fatigue and frustration set in, and your pain increases. This can keep you from doing other things that are equally, if not more, important, such as spending time with family and friends or having quiet time for yourself.

The opposite isn't any better — avoiding all activity and spending hours lying around the house. The isolation this lifestyle produces causes you to focus only on your pain, and it reduces your ability and desire to take part in physical and social activities.

So what is the answer? It's a day that includes a healthy balance — time for work, socializing with family and friends, hobbies, recreation, exercise, relaxation, spirituality, and self-care. Achieving such a balance can be difficult, especially when you first get started. You may have a lot of commitments and responsibilities, and it isn't easy to change old habits.

Instead of drastically altering your daily routine so that it feels uncomfortable, take it one small step at a time. Each week, try to incorporate several small changes, starting with a few routine tasks. Instead of looking at your email over breakfast, enjoy a cup of coffee and the newspaper. Rather than sit at home alone and watch TV, join a community or church group. Over time, you'll achieve a healthy balance.

An unbalanced day

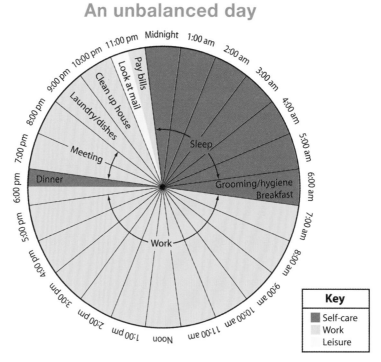

Key
- Self-care
- Work
- Leisure

A balanced day

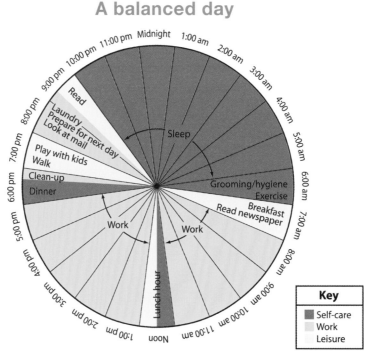

Key
- Self-care
- Work
- Leisure

Learning to balance your day

Think of how you spend a typical weekday. Does it include a balance of activities? The top circle on the opposite page shows imbalance. Work consumes most of this person's daytime hours, leaving little time for other activities. The bottom example shows a more balanced day that includes time for exercise, leisure activities and relaxation. A healthy balance incorporates time for being productive, as well as resting and having fun.

During the week and on the weekends, try not to spend a disproportionate amount of time on any one activity, such as more than eight hours working. Instead, aim to include a variety of activities in your day to achieve a healthy balance. On the weekends, it's OK to incorporate more leisure and self-care activities into your day.

Putting time on your side

For many people, an important step to balancing their day is learning to use time more efficiently. Juggling work, household tasks and social activities can consume large amounts of your day. Procrastination, perfectionism or overcommitting yourself can make time management even more difficult. Taking charge of your time can have a significant impact on how you feel and how much energy you have.

Following are some strategies that can help you use your time more effectively:

Plan
Schedule your day so that you have time for the things you need to do and those you want to do. Write down all of your activities — work and leisure — in a daily planner, or use a calendar on your smartphone. Then frequently refer to your planner or calendar to make sure you stay on track.

It may also be helpful to place a calendar near your telephone to mark down all of your events and appointments so that they don't come as a surprise and to avoid doubling up on commitments. Using a planner doesn't require rigid scheduling. Rather, it simply provides a framework so that you can control and be more aware of how you spend your time.

Recognize patterns
Notice when you waste time — such as staying in bed too long or excessively surfing the Internet — and

Daily planner

Planning your day can help you achieve a healthier balance to your daily routine. Include a mix of work, rest, exercise, relaxation and social activities. If you have trouble fitting everything in, ask yourself: What do I have to do today? What would best be done today? What do I want to do today?

Day & date: Thursday, May 10

	I plan to	I did
6:00 a.m.	Exercise, eat breakfast	Exercised, ate breakfast
7:00 a.m.	Clean up and leave for work	Got ready and went to work
8:00 a.m.	Work on letters from yesterday	Letters
9:00 a.m.	Complete letters	Letters, worked on meeting agenda
10:00 a.m.	Take a break, start work on new files	Agenda, took 10-minute walk
11:00 a.m.	New files	Started new files
Noon	Meet Susan for lunch, relax	Lunch with Susan, breathing exercises
1:00 p.m.	Continue work on files	New files
2:00 p.m.	Department meeting	Meeting
3:00 p.m.	Take a break, complete files	Meeting follow-up, took coffee break
4:00 p.m.	Make phone calls, other details	Phone calls, email, memos
5:00 p.m.	Go home, rest, ride bike	Went home, rested, rode bike
6:00 p.m.	Prepare and eat dinner	Dinner
7:00 p.m.	Do laundry and iron	Laundry, rested
8:00 p.m.	Visit with spouse	Visited with Jim, ironing
9:00 p.m.	Relaxation exercises, rest	Looked at mail, did some yoga
10:00 p.m.	Read book, go to bed	Read book and went to bed
11:00 p.m.	Sleep	Slept

Daily planner

Make photocopies of this page and use the planner to schedule your day. You can plan a day at a time or make your plans for several days. Each day, write down what you actually did and compare it with your plan. If you find that scheduling your day helps you achieve your goals and live a more balanced life, then continue to do so.

Day & date:

	I plan to	I did
6:00 a.m.		
7:00 a.m.		
8:00 a.m.		
9:00 a.m.		
10:00 a.m.		
11:00 a.m.		
Noon		
1:00 p.m.		
2:00 p.m.		
3:00 p.m.		
4:00 p.m.		
5:00 p.m.		
6:00 p.m.		
7:00 p.m.		
8:00 p.m.		
9:00 p.m.		
10:00 p.m.		
11:00 p.m.		

avoid these time wasters. Find ways to make that time more productive. For example, during your daily bus commute or while waiting for a doctor's appointment, you might work on your weekly grocery list or balance your checkbook.

Prioritize

If you're involved in many activities that are competing for your time, decide which are the most important and let go of the rest. Be aware that another person's priority doesn't have to be your priority. There are times when your needs come before the needs of others. The consequence of not taking care of yourself often is increased pain.

Delegate

On days when you have more to do than you can handle, seek help. Asking for assistance, or allowing others to take responsibility for certain things, doesn't indicate a character weakness. To the contrary, delegating is an example of time and energy management. You may delegate all or part of it. To decrease your stress, let go of the task both physically and mentally.

Evaluate

Think about your day. Are your expectations regarding the number of tasks you can complete realistic? If you consistently have too many activities left uncompleted at the end of the day, you may be overscheduling your time.

Educate

Discuss your time needs with those who rely on you the most. If family members, friends or co-workers make unreasonable demands on your time, explain that to stay active and healthy you need to pace yourself and that you're making a conscious effort to live a balanced life.

Becoming more organized

Organization is very important to a healthy lifestyle. It can save you time so that you can incorporate more activities into your day. Organization also helps conserve energy.

Think before you act

Before you begin a task, gather all of the items you'll need or make a list. For example, keep all of your cleaning supplies in one bucket to avoid multiple trips up and down the stairs. Make a list before you run errands to avoid wasted time and additional trips.

Keep commonly used items handy

Organize your work areas at home and at your job so that those items you

Taking time for leisure

People living with chronic pain have a tendency to either abandon all leisure activities or participate in strenuous recreational events regardless of the consequences. Neither approach is good.

You want your day to include some leisure activity, be it active recreation (sports, outings, travel), quiet recreation (hobbies, crafts, reading) or socialization (visiting, making phone calls, attending parties).

Leisure activities are beneficial to your health for many reasons. They reduce stress, enhance self-esteem and confidence, provide fun and enjoyment, and create a distraction from your pain.

The key is to include the right amount of leisure in your day — not too much or too little. It's also good to space your leisure activities throughout the day: Maybe play a short round of golf in the morning, have coffee with friends in the afternoon and read a book in the evening.

As with many other aspects of learning to manage chronic pain, moderation is key. You also want to participate in leisure activities that you enjoy and that are relaxing. If that morning round of golf leaves you frustrated and worsens your pain, you might want to look for another activity.

frequently use are close at hand. This can save you unnecessary bending or reaching. At home, this might include keeping your spoons and spatulas next to the stove, and bowls, kettles and pans within easy reach. In the garage, keep wrenches, screwdrivers and other frequently used items by your workbench.

Reduce clutter
Searching for items takes both time and energy. Organize your work spaces, as well as your drawers and closets, so that you can easily find what you need. Try not to let housework and paperwork pile up. And keep frequently used items, such as your phone and car keys, in the same spot.

Practicing moderation

Moderation involves how much, how long or how fast you do things to avoid overdoing or underdoing activities during your day. By moderating activities, you can improve your ability to accomplish daily and weekly tasks without increasing pain levels or fatigue. To practice moderation:

Break apart lengthy tasks

Lengthy activities often deplete your energy and may increase your pain. Instead of spending all day Saturday planting your garden, spend an hour or two in the garden over three or four days. Another example is to divide a 10-hour car trip to visit relatives into two days instead of one. Get out and stretch every 90 minutes or 90 miles.

Alternate activities

Mix activities that require a lot of effort with those that require little energy. After doing some vacuuming, sit down and fold laundry. After mowing the lawn, read or watch a movie.

Prioritize tasks

Note those times of the day when you have the most energy. Plan your priority tasks — those chores you "have to" get done — during these times.

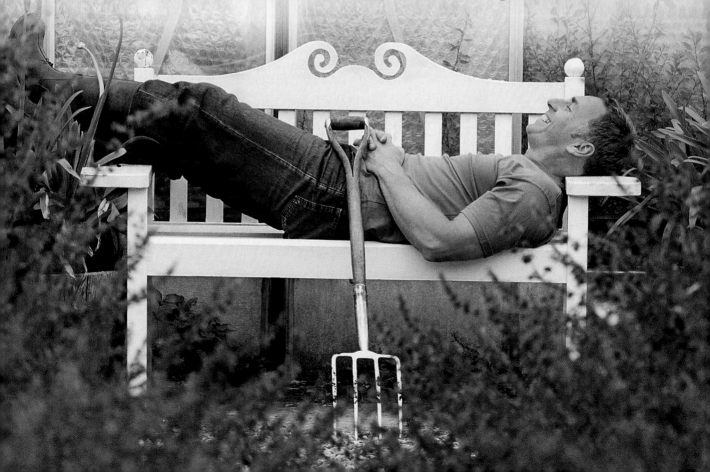

Don't hold your breath

If you've been in an exercise class, you may have heard your instructor say, "Don't forget to breathe." And you may have said to yourself, "Of course I'm breathing." But there are different ways to breathe.

When you're concentrating on an activity such as exercising or struggling with a task such as opening a jar lid, it's common to hold your breath. And often, you don't even realize that you're doing it. When you hold your breath, however, you limit oxygen to your muscles when they need it the most. Because your muscles can't perform to their capacity without adequate oxygen, you become more easily fatigued.

To keep from holding your breath, exhale when you exert the most energy, such as twisting a jar lid or lifting a heavy box from the floor. Your body will naturally respond by breathing in.

Take frequent rest breaks
How often you should take a break depends on the activity. You may find that you can do some activities, such as working at your computer, for 30 minutes to an hour before you need a break. More strenuous tasks, such as mowing the lawn or cleaning the house, may require a break every 10 to 20 minutes. It's important to take a break before you become fatigued.

Work at a moderate pace
Instead of rushing to complete a task, take your time and work at a comfortable speed — one at which you feel like you're exerting yourself but not overdoing it. You expend twice as much energy when you work at a fast pace compared with a moderate one. It may take you a little longer to get the job done, but in the end you'll feel better.

Change the frequency of tasks
Some tasks may be less fatiguing if you break them up and do them more often. For example, rather than spending an entire day on Saturday doing laundry, and becoming worn out in the process, spread out the laundry throughout the week.

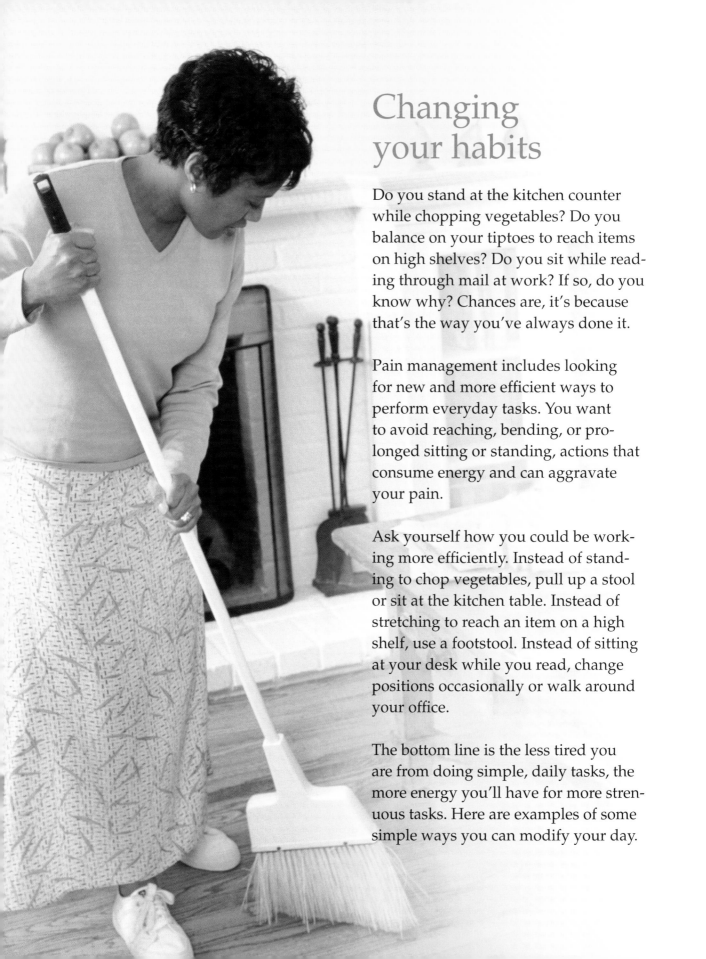

Changing your habits

Do you stand at the kitchen counter while chopping vegetables? Do you balance on your tiptoes to reach items on high shelves? Do you sit while reading through mail at work? If so, do you know why? Chances are, it's because that's the way you've always done it.

Pain management includes looking for new and more efficient ways to perform everyday tasks. You want to avoid reaching, bending, or prolonged sitting or standing, actions that consume energy and can aggravate your pain.

Ask yourself how you could be working more efficiently. Instead of standing to chop vegetables, pull up a stool or sit at the kitchen table. Instead of stretching to reach an item on a high shelf, use a footstool. Instead of sitting at your desk while you read, change positions occasionally or walk around your office.

The bottom line is the less tired you are from doing simple, daily tasks, the more energy you'll have for more strenuous tasks. Here are examples of some simple ways you can modify your day.

While getting dressed

- Gather all articles of clothing.
- Sit down to put on your clothes.
- Place your foot on a chair or stool when tying your shoes.
- Avoid clothes that button or tie in the back.

In the kitchen

- Bend your knees, not your back, to reach items on lower shelves.
- Place one foot on a footstool or low shelf when standing for long periods, and alternate your feet.
- Organize your cupboards so that frequently used items are within easy reach.
- Store heavy items at waist level where they're easily accessible.
- Use electrical appliances when possible, such as an electric mixer or can opener.
- Choose quick and easy recipes or double recipes and freeze extra portions for another day's meal.

Around the house

- Use a long-handled duster for hard-to-reach corners and a long-handled mop to clean your floors.

- Use your legs, not your arm, to move the vacuum cleaner.
- Instead of bending over, sit on a stool to remove laundry from your dryer. Sort your laundry on a table instead of the floor.
- Position your bed so that you have access to it from three sides. When making your bed, get on your knees to tuck in bed sheets and blankets. Instead of lifting the mattress, push the sheets and blankets between the mattress and box spring.

When outdoors

- Use a wheeled cart to move heavy items.
- Mow your lawn with a self-propelled mower.
- Purchase power tools, such as a nail driver and screwdriver.
- Use tools or assistive devices that reduce strain on your joints, such as garden or yard tools with enlarged grips.
- Use a long-handled rake or hoe to avoid bending.
- Bag or mulch leaves instead of rake them.
- Bend your knees when shoveling snow, and use your legs to slide the snow and lift the load. Use a small, lightweight shovel.

Moving your body wisely

Changing how you perform daily activities may be required to use your muscles and joints correctly. Proper body mechanics begin with good posture. When you stand or sit, keep your shoulders and neck relaxed and your spine aligned properly.

If you sit for prolonged periods, occasionally elevate your legs by placing your feet on a footstool. Also change positions to shift your weight. This helps divert stress to different muscles. The same strategies apply to prolonged standing. Shift your weight to change positions and use a footstool.

Here are examples of proper ways to move your body when performing basic tasks.

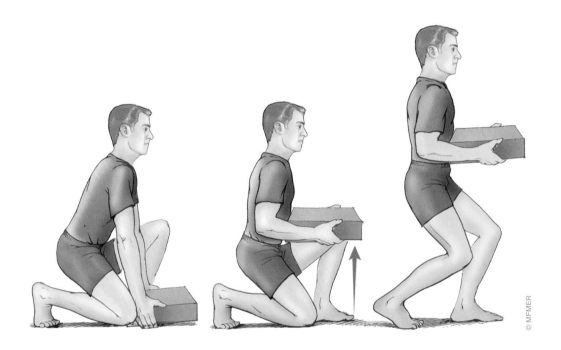

When lifting

Follow the basic steps for kneeling (see page 199). Get close to the object you're going to lift. If the object is heavy, lift it first to your bent knee. Then lift the object using your leg muscles. As you rise from the floor, keep your head facing forward to protect your back. Carry the object close to your body at about waist level. Turn by pivoting your feet. Don't twist at your waist.

When using long-handled tools

Stand with one foot forward and shift your weight forward and backward on each foot. During the forward stroke, shift your body weight to your forward foot. When you pull back, shift your weight to your back foot. Use arm and leg movements instead of back movements. Avoid overreaching and twisting. Use long, smooth strokes and reposition your feet if needed. Occasionally switch hands.

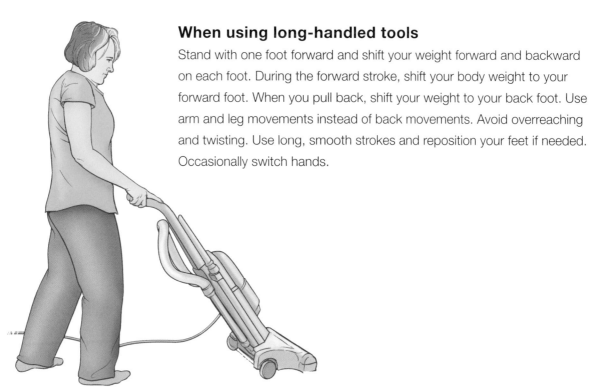

When reaching

Stand close to the object you're retrieving. Avoid excessive arching and twisting of your back. Place one foot forward as close to the object as possible. Grasp the object and bring it to the edge of the shelf by shifting your body weight to your back foot. Slowly lower the object to waist level, using your arms. Keep the object as close to you as possible.

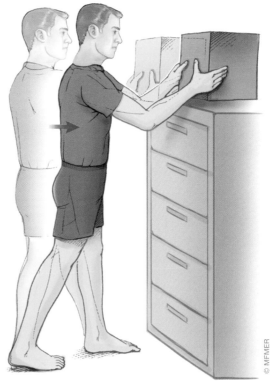

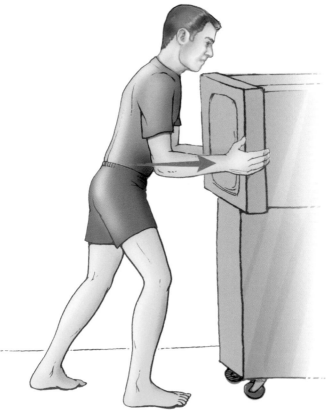

When pushing

Keep your feet apart and your back straight. Bend your knees but not your back. Walk slowly, using your legs to push the object ahead of you.

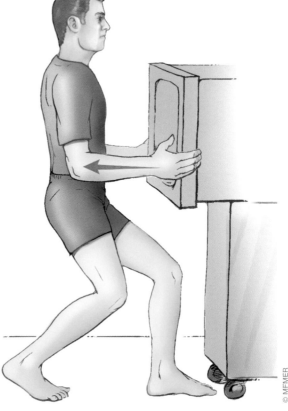

When pulling

Keep your feet apart and your back straight. Bend your knees but not your back. Slowly walk backward, using your whole body weight, not just your arms or back, to pull the object. If possible, push the object rather than pull it.

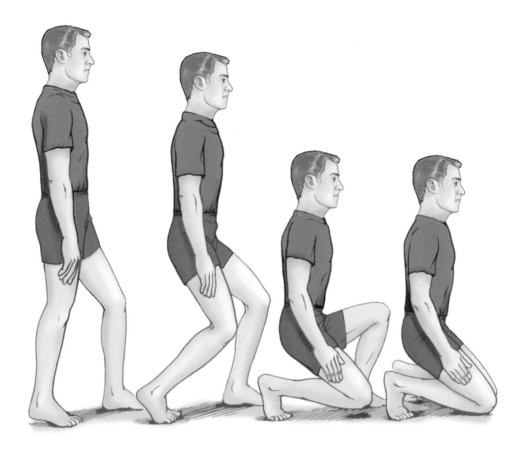

When kneeling

Keep your feet 8 to 12 inches (shoulder-width) apart. Place one foot forward and lower your body to one knee, keeping your weight on the balls of your feet. If you need to, place your hands on your thighs or hold on to a stable object to help you move in and out of a kneeling position. Keep your back straight. To progress to full kneeling, lower yourself until both knees are on the floor, and sit back on your heels. Reverse the process to stand.

Get smart

Here are examples of daily living goals that follow the SMART formula:

Goal: Spend fewer hours at work or doing work activities at home
When I want to achieve it: Four weeks
How I'm going to do it: Try to leave the office at 5:30 each day, don't stay to "finish up" a task, try not to bring work home
How I'm going to measure it: Record each day in my journal how many hours I spent at work or on work-related tasks at home

Goal: Find time for relaxation in my busy schedule
When I want to achieve it: By the end of the week
How I'm going to do it: After dinner perform 15 minutes of diaphragmatic breathing in the living room with the TV turned off
How I'm going to measure it: Each day, in my journal or on a chart, rate my tension level before and after relaxation to track my progress and hold myself accountable

Chapter 14

Caring for yourself

L iving well with chronic pain isn't just about managing the pain. It's about caring for your overall health so that you can enjoy life to its fullest.

Becoming more physically active, reducing stress and learning how to relax are discussed in separate chapters. This chapter focuses on other factors, such as sleep, weight and diet, alcohol and smoking, sexuality, and your spiritual needs, which can help you stay active and productive.

Getting a good night's sleep

Sleep refreshes you. It improves your attitude and gives you energy for physical activity and to fight off fatigue and stress. It also boosts your immune system, reducing your risk of illness.

If you aren't sleeping well, it may be because your pain is keeping you from falling asleep or is waking you up at night. Other factors that can interfere with sleep are:

- Stress
- Stimulant medications
- Anxiety
- Regular use of sleeping pills
- Depression
- Alcohol
- Lack of physical activity
- Poor sleep habits
- Change in your environment

To improve your sleep, it's important to recognize those factors that may be contributing to your restless nights and find ways to deal with them.

Stages of sleep

During the night, you cycle from light sleep to deep sleep and back to light sleep. Most people typically experience four to six sleep cycles, moving from one stage to another with each cycle lasting about 90 minutes.

There are two types of sleep — non-rapid eye movement (NREM) and rapid eye movement (REM). Your nightly journey begins as you pass into stage one of NREM sleep, a light sleep. During NREM sleep, your brain activity and body functions slow. Later stages of NREM sleep, called delta sleep or deep sleep, are the most restful. In these stages, brain waves are large and slow, and you're more difficult to awaken.

REM, or dream, sleep occurs about one and a half to two hours after you fall asleep. In this sleep stage, brain activity increases and your eyes move rapidly behind your closed eyelids, hence the name. Your body, however, typically doesn't move. You do more thinking, in the form of dreaming, in this stage.

Sleep is important, because it restores you mentally, emotionally and physically. Lack of sleep affects not only your energy level but also your social and mental functioning. Losing sleep can cause difficulty with concentration and increased irritability. Insomnia also may be related to depression. In addition, studies have also found you're more prone to weight gain if you don't get enough sleep.

You want to develop a healthy sleep schedule — a sleep routine in which you get enough sleep to help you function well, but not too much so that it affects the quality of your sleep.

Tips to help you sleep better

Before bed, take time to relax. Doing so will help you sleep better. Some of the many activities that promote relaxation include:

- Deep breathing and muscle relaxation
- Taking a warm bath
- Having a light snack
- Reading
- Listening to soothing music
- Writing in your journal

Relaxation helps reduce your pain so that you can fall asleep more easily. It also helps you achieve more restful sleep. Here are other suggestions that may help you sleep better:

- **Establish regular sleep hours.** Go to bed and wake up at the same time each day — even on weekends.
- **Limit your time in bed.** Too much sleep can promote shallow, unrestful sleep. In addition, spending too much time in bed also disrupts sleep. Nine out of 10 people with insomnia stay in bed longer than necessary.
- **Don't try to sleep.** The harder you try, the more awake you'll become. Read or watch television until you become drowsy and fall asleep naturally.
- **Limit bedroom activities.** Save your bedroom for sleep and sex. Don't watch TV or take your work materials to bed.
- **Watch what you eat.** A light snack may help you relax before sleeping. However, avoid heavy meals and fluids or foods that stimulate stomach acid production, which could cause heartburn or irritate your esophagus.
- **Avoid or limit caffeine, alcohol and nicotine.** Caffeine and nicotine can keep you from falling asleep. Alcohol may make you sleepy, but it often causes unrestful sleep and frequent awakenings during the night.
- **Minimize interruptions.** Close your bedroom door or create a subtle background noise, such as that from a fan, to muffle other noises. Drink less before you go to bed so that you won't have to get up during the night to go to the bathroom.
- **Get comfy.** Make sure you have a bed that's comfortable and keep your bedroom temperature at a comfortably cool level.
- **Hide the clock.** A visible indicator of how long you've been unable to sleep may make you needlessly anxious. Place clocks where they aren't visible or within reach.
- **Keep active.** Regular physical activity helps you sleep more soundly. Try to get at least 30 minutes of physical activity daily, preferably five to six hours before bedtime. Also keep busy throughout the day. Boredom promotes restless sleep.
- **Avoid or limit naps.** Naps can make it harder to fall asleep at night.
- **Schedule worry time.** Your bedroom is your sanctuary for sleep. Don't take your worries to bed with you. Before you go to bed, take time to address your worries and think of ways you might solve them.
- **Check your medications.** Ask your doctor if your medications might be contributing to your difficulty sleeping. Also check over-the-counter products that you're taking to see if they contain caffeine or other stimulants, such as pseudoephedrine.

To nap, or not?

The urge for a midday snooze is built into your body's biological clock. It generally hits between 1 p.m. and 4 p.m., when your body temperature naturally dips slightly. Napping shouldn't be viewed as a substitute for a full night's sleep. You shouldn't nap if you have trouble sleeping at night. However, if you find that a nap refreshes you and doesn't interfere with nighttime sleep, it's OK to take one, provided you:

Keep it short. Thirty minutes is ideal. Naps longer than one to two hours are more likely to interfere with your nighttime sleep.

Take a midafternoon nap. Naps at this time of the day produce a physically invigorating slumber.

Simply rest awhile, if you can't sleep. Lie down and keep your mind on something relaxing.

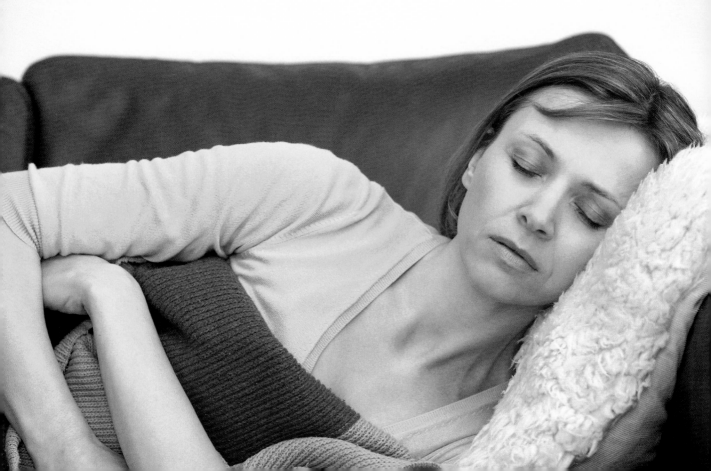

What about medications?

If you're having trouble sleeping, your doctor may prescribe a sleep medication until other steps to improve your sleep and control your pain have time to take effect.

The downfall of many prescription and over-the-counter sleep medications — and why it's often recommended that they not be used long-term — is that the medicines generally don't allow you to experience all phases of sleep.

Sleep medications can also lose their effectiveness and cause side effects, including dry mouth, next-day drowsiness and physical dependence. Plus, over time, the drugs can actually make it more difficult for you to get restful sleep.

For sleep difficulties associated with chronic pain, antidepressant medications are often prescribed (see page 108). A side effect of some antidepressants is drowsiness. When taken before bed, they can help you sleep.

Another treatment tool that's gaining in popularity is cognitive behavioral therapy. Cognitive behavioral therapy is a structured program that helps you identify and replace negative thoughts and unhealthy behaviors that cause or worsen sleep problems with healthy habits that promote sound sleep.

Instead of just treating your symptoms, this type of treatment is intended to help you overcome the underlying causes of your sleep problems.

Controlling your weight

Maintaining a healthy weight reduces your risk of illnesses such as cardiovascular disease, high blood pressure and diabetes. It's also easier to manage your pain when you're not overweight. That's because excessive weight saps your energy level, increases stress on muscles and joints, and decreases your flexibility.

It's not necessary that you become thin. But losing even a few pounds may help reduce your level of pain, as well as your blood sugar and cholesterol levels.

Is your weight healthy?

Three do-it-yourself evaluations can tell you if your weight is healthy or whether you could benefit from weight loss.

What's your BMI?

You can determine your body mass index (BMI) by finding your height and weight on this chart. A BMI of 18.5 to 24.9 is considered the healthiest. People with a BMI under 18.5 are considered underweight. People with a BMI between 25 and 29.9 are considered overweight. People with a BMI of 30 or greater are considered obese.

	Normal		Overweight					Obese				
BMI	19	24	25	26	27	28	29	30	35	40	45	50
Height							Weight in pounds					
4'10"	91	115	119	124	129	134	138	143	167	191	215	239
4'11"	94	119	124	128	133	138	143	148	173	198	222	247
5'0"	97	123	128	133	138	143	148	153	179	204	230	255
5'1"	100	127	132	137	143	148	153	158	185	211	238	264
5'2"	104	131	136	142	147	153	158	164	191	218	246	273
5'3"	107	135	141	146	152	158	163	169	197	225	254	282
5'4"	110	140	145	151	157	163	169	174	204	232	262	291
5'5"	114	144	150	156	162	168	174	180	210	240	270	300
5'6"	118	148	155	161	167	173	179	186	216	247	278	309
5'7"	121	153	159	166	172	178	185	191	223	255	287	319
5'8"	125	158	164	171	177	184	190	197	230	262	295	328
5'9"	128	162	169	176	182	189	196	203	236	270	304	338
5'10"	132	167	174	181	188	195	202	209	243	278	313	348
5'11"	136	172	179	186	193	200	208	215	250	286	322	358
6'0"	140	177	184	191	199	206	213	221	258	294	331	368
6'1"	144	182	189	197	204	212	219	227	265	302	340	378
6'2"	148	186	194	202	210	218	225	233	272	311	350	389
6'3"	152	192	200	208	216	224	232	240	279	319	359	399
6'4"	156	197	205	213	221	230	238	246	287	328	369	410

Source: National Institutes of Health (NIH), 1998

Asians with a BMI of 23 or higher may have an increased risk of health problems.

Body mass index

Body mass index (BMI) is a formula that considers your weight and your height in determining whether you have a healthy or unhealthy percentage of total body fat. It's a better measurement of health risks related to your weight than using your bathroom scale or standard height-and-weight tables.

To determine your BMI, locate your height on the chart on the previous page and follow it across until you reach the weight nearest yours. Look at the top of the column for the BMI rating. If your weight is less than the weight nearest yours, your BMI may be slightly less. If your weight is greater than the weight nearest yours, your BMI may be slightly greater. A BMI of 18.5 to 24.9 is considered healthy. A BMI of 25 to 29.9 signifies overweight, and a BMI of 30 or more indicates obesity.

Waist circumference

This measurement indicates where most of your body fat is located. People who carry most of their weight around their waists may be referred to as apple-like. Those who carry most of their weight below their waists, around their hips and thighs, are described as pear-like.

Generally, it's better to have a pear shape than to have an apple shape.

That's because fat around your abdomen is associated with a greater risk of cardiovascular and other weight-related diseases.

To determine whether you're carrying too much weight around your abdomen, measure your waist circumference. Find the highest point on each of your hipbones and measure across your abdomen just above those points. A measurement of more than 40 inches (102 centimeters) in men and 35 inches (89 centimeters) in women signifies increased health risks, especially if you have a BMI of 25 or more.

Personal and family history

An evaluation of your medical history, along with that of your family, is equally important in determining whether your weight is healthy. Answer these questions:

- Do you have a health condition, such as arthritis or back pain, that would benefit from weight loss?
- Do you have a family history of a weight-related illness, such as diabetes, high blood pressure or high cholesterol?
- Have you gained considerable weight since high school? Weight gain in adulthood is associated with increased health risks.

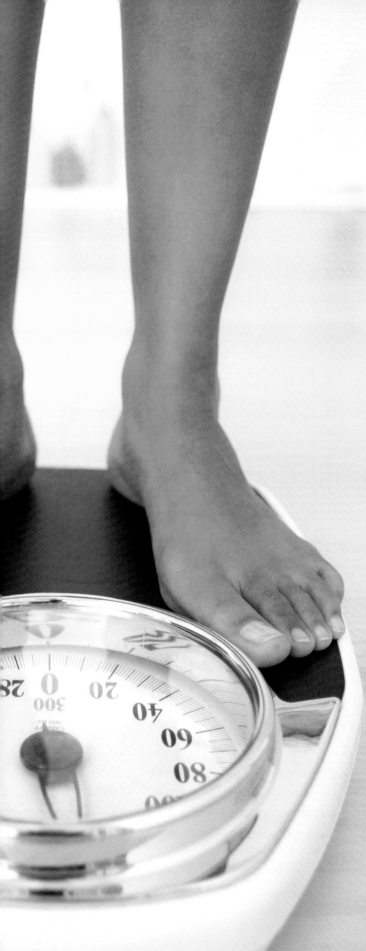

- Do you smoke cigarettes, have more than two alcoholic drinks a day or live with considerable stress? In combination with these behaviors, excess weight can have greater health implications.

Adding up the results

If your BMI shows that you aren't overweight, you're not carrying too much weight around your abdomen, and you answered no to all of the personal or family history questions, there's probably no health advantage to changing your weight — it's healthy. However, it's important for you to maintain good eating and exercise habits to help keep you from gaining weight as you age.

If your BMI is between 25 and 29.9, your waist circumference exceeds healthy guidelines, or you answered yes to at least one personal and family health question, you might benefit from losing a few pounds. Discuss your weight with your doctor during your next visit.

If your BMI is 30 or more, losing weight will improve your overall health and energy level and reduce your risk of future illness. You should try to lose weight.

Losing weight successfully

The best way to lose weight safely and keep it off permanently is through lifestyle changes. There are many products and programs that promise to help you shed pounds, but they aren't always safe or effective. Once you go off the diet, you almost always gain the weight back again. To increase your chances of being successful:

- **Make a commitment.** You must be motivated to lose weight because it's what you want, not what someone else wants you to do. Only you can lose weight. But that doesn't mean you have to do everything alone. Your doctor or a registered dietitian can help you plan how best to lose weight.
- **Think positively.** Don't dwell on what you're giving up to lose weight. Instead, concentrate on what you're gaining. Instead of thinking, "I really miss eating a doughnut for breakfast," tell yourself, "I feel a lot better when I eat whole-wheat toast and cereal in the morning."
- **Set a realistic goal.** Don't aim for a weight that's unrealistic. If you've always been overweight, aim for a weight that will help reduce pressure on your joints and muscles and improve your energy level. Studies show that losing even 10 percent of what you weigh can improve your health and sense of well-being. Because weight can fluctuate considerably over the short term due to a variety of factors, your goals should include behaviors that are within your control.
- **Accept that healthy weight loss is slow and steady.** A good weight-loss plan generally involves losing no more than 1 to 2 pounds a week. Set weekly or monthly goals that allow you to check off your successes. Reward yourself when you meet a goal.
- **Know your habits.** Ask yourself if you tend to eat when you're bored, angry, tired, anxious, depressed or socially pressured. If you do, before eating anything, ask yourself if you really want it. If you're feeling stressed, upset or angry, direct that energy constructively. Instead of eating, practice a relaxation technique or take a long, brisk walk.
- **Don't starve yourself.** Many people try to lose weight by consuming only 1,000 to 1,500 calories a day. Cutting calories to fewer than 1,200 if you're a woman or 1,400 if you're a man doesn't provide enough food to keep you satisfied. When you're hungry, your risk of overeating or eating unhealthy foods is greater.

Plus, too few calories promotes temporary loss of fluids and loss of healthy muscle, instead of permanent loss of fat.

- **Get and stay active.** Eating more healthfully will help you lose weight, but adding 30 minutes of moderate activity most days of the week will help increase your rate of weight loss. Physical activity is the most important factor related to long-term weight loss. It promotes loss of body fat and development of muscle. These changes in body composition raise the rate at which you burn calories, making it easier to maintain your weight loss. Only you will know how much you can exercise. Pain may impose limits on the types of exercise you do. However, exercise may also relieve pain and stiffness.

- **Think lifelong.** It's not enough to eat healthy foods and exercise

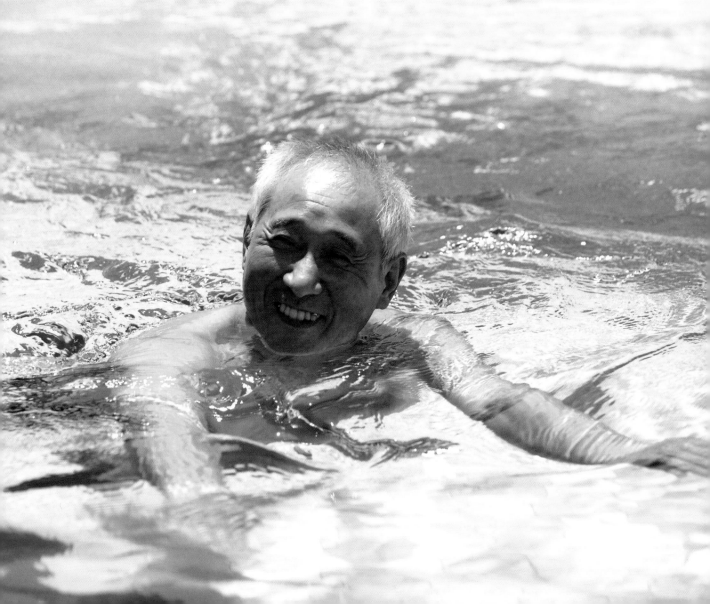

for a few weeks or even several months. As with other strategies for managing your pain, you have to incorporate these new behaviors into your life.

Eating better

Food can't control your pain. But a nutritionally balanced diet can improve the way you feel. In addition to helping you lose weight, eating a variety of foods gives you energy and a sense of well-being.

Experts agree that the best way to increase nutrients in your diet and limit fat and calories is to eat more plant-based foods. Plant foods — fruits, vegetables and foods made from whole grains — contain beneficial vitamins, minerals, fibers and health-enhancing compounds called phytochemicals. By emphasizing plant foods in your diet, you increase consumption of many naturally healthy compounds.

For good health and to achieve and maintain a healthy weight, you want to eat a healthy balance of foods each day. A tool that can help you eat well is the Mayo Clinic Healthy Weight Pyramid (see page 212). The pyramid illustrates the types and amounts of food you

need to eat every day from each of the six represented food groups.

Vegetables

Eat at least four servings of vegetables every day. Vegetables are naturally low in calories, and almost all are fat-free. They provide vitamins, minerals, fiber and phytochemicals.

Fresh vegetables are best, but frozen vegetables are good, too. Most canned vegetables are high in sodium, which is used as a preservative in the canning process. Excessive sodium can increase blood pressure in some people. If you eat canned vegetables, select those indicating that no sodium has been added or the sodium is reduced.

Fruits

You can also eat fruit in unlimited quantities, with the exception of dried fruit and fruit juices, which are high in calories. Try to include at least three servings of fruit daily.

Fruit contains little or no fat, and it provides many beneficial nutrients and phytochemicals. Fresh fruit is generally best. It makes a great snack. If you get the urge to snack between meals or you have a sweet tooth, keep a bowl of fresh fruit nearby. Frozen fruits with no added sugar and fruits

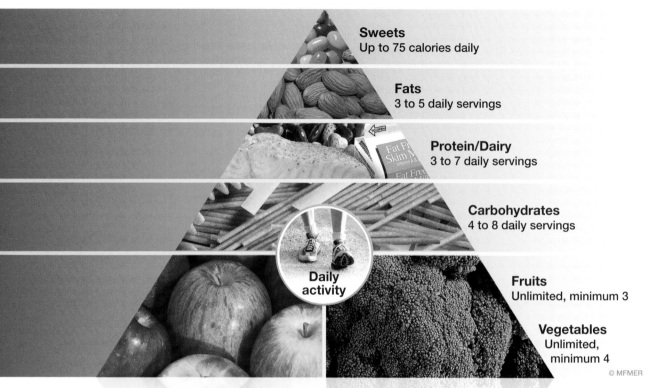

Sweets
Up to 75 calories daily

Fats
3 to 5 daily servings

Protein/Dairy
3 to 7 daily servings

Carbohydrates
4 to 8 daily servings

Daily activity

Fruits
Unlimited, minimum 3

Vegetables
Unlimited, minimum 4

© MFMER

Mayo Clinic Healthy Weight Pyramid
See your doctor before you begin any healthy weight plan

canned in water or their own juices are acceptable alternatives.

Carbohydrates

Carbohydrates include grain products, such as cereals, breads, rice and pasta, and starchy vegetables, such as corn, potatoes and some types of squash.

Along with vegetables and fruits, carbohydrates should form the foundation of your daily diet. Whenever possible, select whole-grain foods over refined products. Whole grains contain bran and germ, which add fiber. Whole grains are also important sources of vitamins and minerals.

Some carbohydrates, such as croissants, chips, crackers and dessert breads, are high in fat and calories. Make sure you read the nutrition label. Bread, pasta and most plain cereals are fairly low in fat and calories. It's what you put on these low-fat foods — whole milk, cream, or spreads and sauces made from fats, oils or cheese — that adds calories.

Protein and dairy

Protein is an essential nutrient that helps maintain body tissues, such as skin, bone and muscle. Protein is found in a variety of foods, including milk, yogurt, cheese, eggs, meat, poultry, fish and legumes (beans, dried peas and lentils). Most Americans eat far more protein than they need, especially those products that are high in fat and calories, such as meat.

Make sure to include low-fat or fat-free milk or milk products (yogurt and cheese) in your daily diet. Milk, yogurt and cheese are major sources of calcium and vitamin D. Calcium helps keep your bones healthy and reduces your risk of osteoporosis, a disease that reduces bone density and makes your bones brittle. Adequate vitamin D is also important to bone health.

Always try to select fat-free or low-fat varieties of protein, such as poultry (without skin), fish, lean meats, legumes, skim milk and low-fat cheeses.

Fats

A small amount of fat in your diet is necessary to help your body function, but most people consume far more fat than they need. Foods high in fat include products produced mainly from oils, butter, margarine, salad dressing or mayonnaise. An easy way to reduce fat in your diet is to reduce the amount of oil, butter and margarine you add

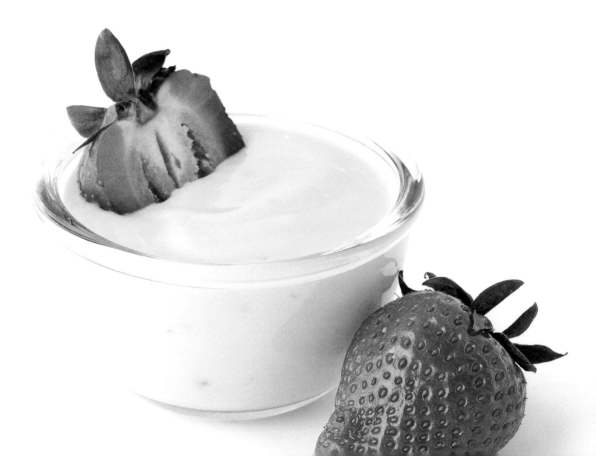

Moderate drinking means no more than one alcoholic drink each day for women and no more than two alcoholic drinks daily for men.

One drink equals one 12-ounce bottle of beer, one 5-ounce glass of wine or one 1.5-ounce shot glass of 80-proof liquor.

For men age 65 and older, moderate drinking is one drink daily. The amount is less because older individuals typically process alcohol more slowly.

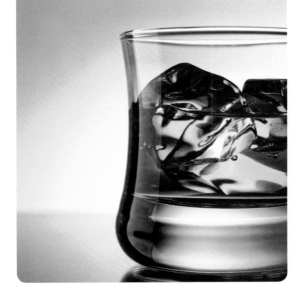

to food when preparing it. Many snack products, such as chips and crackers, also are high in fat.

Healthier fats include those that contain monounsaturated fat, such as olive oil and canola oil. But even these should be eaten sparingly.

Sweets

Sweets such as candy and desserts contain considerable calories, and they offer little in terms of nutrition. Many sweets are also high in fat.

You don't have to give up sweets entirely to eat healthfully, but be smart about your selections and portion sizes. Instead of sugar-sweetened soft drinks, candy bars or pastries, consider water, fresh fruit, low-fat frozen yogurt, angel food cake or reduced-calorie cookies.

Limiting alcohol

The best advice about alcohol is that if you drink, do it in moderation. And if you're taking medication, it might be best not to drink any alcohol.

Alcohol can increase the potency and side effects of many prescription drugs, including pain relievers and antide-

Get smart

Here are some lifestyle goals that follow the SMART formula:

Goal: To sleep at least six hours without awakening
When I want to achieve it: Four weeks
How I'm going to do it: Go to bed at the same time each night; use relaxation techniques before bed; be more active during the day
How I'm going to measure it: In my journal, log how many hours I sleep at night without waking up

Goal: To eat more healthy foods
When I want to achieve it: One week
How I'm going to do it: Eat more fruit and less chips and chocolate; have a vegetable with lunch and dinner; eat less beef
How I'm going to measure it: Buy less junk foods and more healthy food; a couple of times a week write down what I eat

pressants. In addition, regularly combining alcohol with over-the-counter pain relievers, including acetaminophen or nonsteroidal anti-inflammatory drugs (NSAIDs), may increase your risk of liver damage.

Using alcohol to help relieve your pain or to deal with the toll it's causing on you and your family can also lead to dependence and addiction. If you regularly drink more than a moderate amount of alcohol, talk with your doctor about the safest and most successful way to limit or avoid alcohol.

Quitting smoking

There's no question smoking is dangerous to your health. Tobacco smoke contains a multitude of substances that can damage your heart and blood vessels and cause cancer.

Smoking also contributes to chronic pain by increasing fatigue and muscle weakness. Carbon monoxide in tobacco smoke replaces oxygen in your red blood cells. Less oxygen means less energy and fewer nutrients for your body tissues.

Medications to help you stop smoking

Most people use at least one medication when they try to stop smoking, but many find that a combination of medications is the most comfortable and effective approach. Use them according to your doctor's instructions or, in the case of over-the-counter (OTC) medications, according to instructions on the label.

Nicotine replacement products deliver small doses of nicotine to help relieve withdrawal symptoms but don't keep a smoker addicted to the substance. These products are considered temporary aids — usually for several weeks and at most several months. Consult your doctor about tapering off these medications.

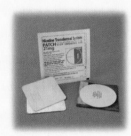

Nicotine patches. Similar to an adhesive bandage, a nicotine patch is placed on your skin and gradually releases nicotine into your body. It's an over-the-counter product and comes in different sizes — the larger the patch, the more nicotine delivered. To minimize skin irritation, rotate the site of the patch and apply an OTC cortisone cream.

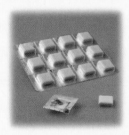

Nicotine gum. This OTC product isn't chewed like normal gum. Bite into the nicotine gum a few times, then "park" it between your cheek and gum and leave it there. The lining of your mouth absorbs the nicotine that the gum releases. Two doses are available — 2 milligrams (mg) and 4 mg. Chew enough gum to relieve your symptoms. You can use up to 20 pieces daily.

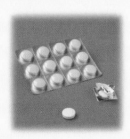

Nicotine lozenges. Nicotine lozenges dissolve in your mouth and, like nicotine gum, deliver nicotine through the lining or your mouth. It looks like a hard candy and releases nicotine as it slowly dissolves in the mouth. Doses are available in 2-mg and 4-mg amounts — the 4-mg lozenge is used by heavier smokers.

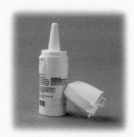

Nicotine nasal spray. You spray this product into your nose with a bottle dispenser. The nicotine is absorbed into your bloodstream through the lining of your nose. The nasal spray delivers nicotine a bit quicker than gum, lozenges or the patch, but not as rapidly as smoking a cigarette. It's often used with nicotine patch therapy or with bupropion medication. The product is available only by prescription.

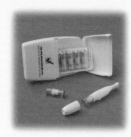

Nicotine inhaler. This device looks like a plastic cigarette that you put to your mouth and puff on, releasing a nicotine vapor into your mouth. Although it's called an inhaler, it doesn't deliver nicotine to the lungs. This product is available only by prescription and the dose is individualized. Using an inhaler also helps smokers who miss the hand-to-mouth ritual that's part of smoking a cigarette.

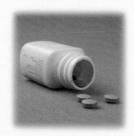

Non-nicotine medications. Bupropion (Zyban) is a nonaddicting, non-nicotine medication approved by the Food and Drug Administration (FDA) as a stop-smoking aid. It's not clear exactly how the drug works. One theory is that bupropion stimulates dopamine, a brain chemical that causes a feel-good response similar to that produced by nicotine and other addictive drugs. Bupropion is available only by prescription.

Varenicline (Chantix) also is approved by the FDA to stop smoking. The medication stimulates the same brain receptors usually activated by the nicotine in tobacco products. Chantix also blocks some of the pleasure you get from smoking, making smoking less rewarding. Nortriptyline (Pamelor) is a tricyclic antidepressant that's been shown to help smokers stop. It increases levels of the brain neurotransmitter norepinephrine. It's used as a second line medication to treat tobacco dependence.

Breaking tobacco's grip

Some people can simply stop and never smoke again. For others, quitting takes several tries and various approaches. Don't let one failed attempt to quit keep you from trying again. You can learn from previous attempts, increasing your chances for being successful in the future. Follow these steps:

- **Do your homework.** That way you'll know what to expect. You may experience physical withdrawal symptoms for at least 10 days. Common symptoms include irritability, anxiety and loss of concentration. Afterward, you may still have the urge to light up in familiar smoking situations, such as after a meal or while driving. These urges are generally brief, but they can be strong. By knowing what to expect and having alternative activities planned, you'll be better prepared to handle the urges. Alternatives might include chewing gum after a meal or snacking on carrot sticks to keep your hands busy.

- **Set a stop date.** For some people, quitting cold turkey works better than cutting down gradually. Carefully select a date to quit smoking. Many smokers choose to quit during vacation or while on a trip when they're away from their usual routines and smoking situations. One reason is that your routine often changes while on vacation. It's easier to break free of smoking rituals when you're away than when you're at work or home.

- **Tell others about your decision.** Having the support of family, friends and co-workers can help you reach your goal more quickly. However, many smokers keep their plans to quit a secret because they don't want to look like a failure if they go back to smoking. Many people try three or more times before they're successful, so don't give up.

- **Start changing your routine.** Before your stop date, cut down on the number of places you smoke. For instance, stop smoking in your car, and smoke in only one room of the house or outside. This approach will help reduce your smoking urges so that you can be more comfortable in those places without smoking.

- **Talk with your doctor about medications.** Nicotine is a highly addictive substance. Withdrawal from nicotine can cause irritability, anxiety and difficulty concentrating. Medications are available that can help lessen withdrawal symptoms and increase your chances of being successful.

- **Take it one day at a time.** On your stop day, quit completely. Each day, focus your attention on remaining tobacco-free.
- **Avoid smoking situations.** Leave the table right after meals if this is the time you used to light up. If you smoked while on the telephone, avoid long phone conversations or talk while doing other things. If you had a favorite smoking chair, avoid it. You'll soon be able to anticipate when the urge to smoke will hit you. Before it hits, start doing something that makes smoking inconvenient, such as washing your car or doing relaxation exercises. Your smoking behavior is deeply ingrained and automatic. You need to anticipate and plan.
- **Time each urge.** Check your watch when a smoking urge hits. Most are short. Once you realize this, it's easier to resist. Tell yourself, "I can make it another few minutes and then the urge will pass."

Expressing your sexuality

Sexuality is a natural and healthy part of living, and a part of your identity as a man or woman. It involves the timeless desire for both physical and emotional intimacy. Sexuality can be expressed through shared interests and companionship, as well as physical contact, including holding hands and sexual intercourse.

When chronic pain invades your life, the pleasures of sexuality often disappear. You may not feel like socializing, sharing your thoughts and feelings, or having close contact. Perhaps you feel your pain has made you less desirable to your partner. Your sleeping arrangement may even have changed. Some people sleep in a spare bedroom or a lounger because they have difficulty getting comfortable or they don't want to keep their partner awake.

In spite of your pain, you can have a healthy and satisfying sexual relationship. It begins with honest communication. You and your partner need to talk about how you feel, what you miss and what you would like from your relationship. You also need to be creative and willing to make changes. That could be as basic as buying a new mattress or a bigger bed so that you don't have to sleep apart, or exploring different ways to express your sexuality.

In all partnerships it takes effort to maintain what's good and to correct what isn't. A healthy sexual relationship can positively affect all aspects of your life, including your physical health, self-esteem, productivity and other relationships.

Becoming more intimate

Start slowly. Before concentrating on improving your sexual relationship, start by spending more time talking. Get to know one another again.

Also look for ways to rekindle your romance. Go on a date, plan a picnic, send flowers or exchange small, personal gifts.

Remind yourself that problems are also opportunities. In your efforts to become more intimate you may discover something about your partner that you otherwise might have missed. The relationship you recover may be even better than the one you had before your pain.

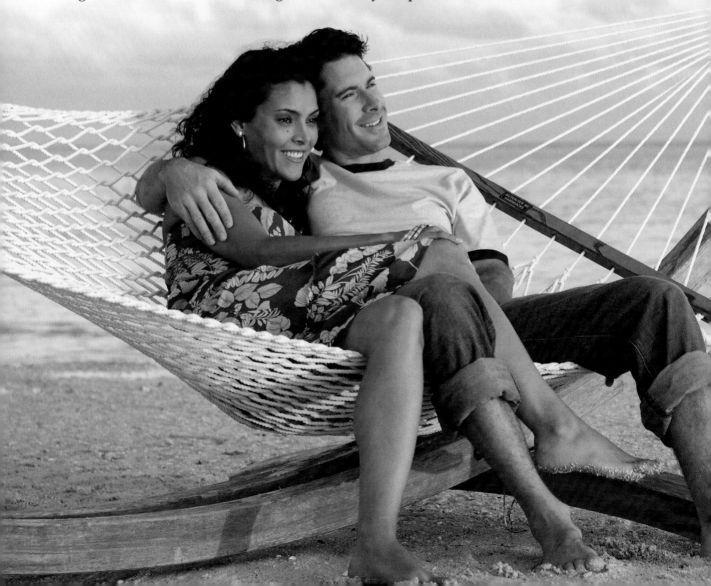

Making love creatively

Sexual intercourse is just one way to satisfy your need for human closeness. Intimacy can be expressed in many different ways.

Touch. Exploring your partner's body through touch is an exciting way to express your sexual feelings. This can include cuddling, fondling, stroking, massaging and kissing. Touch in any form increases feelings of intimacy.

Self-stimulation. Masturbation is a normal and healthy way to fulfill your sexual needs. One partner may use masturbation during mutual sexual activity if the other partner is unable to be very active.

Timing. A change in the time of day you have sexual intercourse may improve your lovemaking. Many people often have higher pain levels in the evening. If this is true for you, you and your partner might try intercourse in the morning or afternoon.

Different positions. Experiment with different positions. Lie side by side, kneel or sit. There are many books and brochures available that describe different ways to have intercourse.

Vibrators and lubricants. A vibrator can add pleasure without physical exertion. If lack of natural lubrication is a problem, over-the-counter lubricants can prevent pain associated with vaginal dryness.

Fears about being intimate

You or your partner may have unspoken fears regarding sexual contact and, because of this, may avoid intimate encounters. Delaying intimacy only increases the anxiety surrounding sexual intercourse. Talking openly with your partner about your fears may help ease them.

Fear of increased pain

It's natural to want to avoid additional pain. And it's common to worry that sexual intercourse will cause you physical pain, especially if your pain is centered in your back, abdomen or pelvis.

Experimenting with different positions and other ways to satisfy your and your partner's sexual needs can help the two of you enjoy intimate encounters (see "Making love creatively" on page 221). Relaxation exercises before and after intercourse also may help reduce fears and manage pain.

Fear of partner rejection

This is a common feeling. You may wonder if your partner is less attracted to you because of your pain. The longer you have these fears, the more difficult it may be to overcome them. Talk openly with your partner about your feelings and fears and encourage your partner to do the same.

Fear of failure to perform

If you're having difficulty becoming sexually aroused, maintaining an erection or achieving an orgasm, talk with your doctor.

Your pain itself, depression, concern over your physical appearance, alcohol and medications all can affect your sexual performance. In addition, many medications, including antidepressants, sedatives and opioids, can reduce your

sexual ability, including making you impotent. If you suspect a medication may be affecting your sexual performance, don't stop taking the drug without first consulting your doctor.

Sometimes, failure to perform is simply a result of stress and anxiety. Patience and understanding can often help you overcome the problem.

Addressing your spiritual needs

The role of spirituality is an important aspect of a person's well-being that's often overlooked. People tend to use the term *spirituality* interchangeably with *religion*. However, the terms aren't necessarily synonymous. Spirituality is as much connected with the spirit and the soul as it is with any specific belief or form of worship. Spirituality is about meaning, values and purpose in life.

Religion may be one way of expressing spirituality, but it's not the only way. For some people, spirituality is feeling in tune with nature and the universe. For still others, spirituality is expressed through music, meditation or art.

For some people, addressing their spiritual needs brings inner peace and added strength to deal with their pain and stress.

Spirituality and healing

Numerous studies have attempted to measure the effect of spirituality on illness and recovery. In reviewing many of these studies, researchers at Georgetown University School of Medicine found at least 80 percent of the studies suggest spiritual beliefs provide health benefits. People who consider themselves to be spiritual generally live longer, recover from illness more quickly, suffer less depression and addiction, and cope better with serious disease.

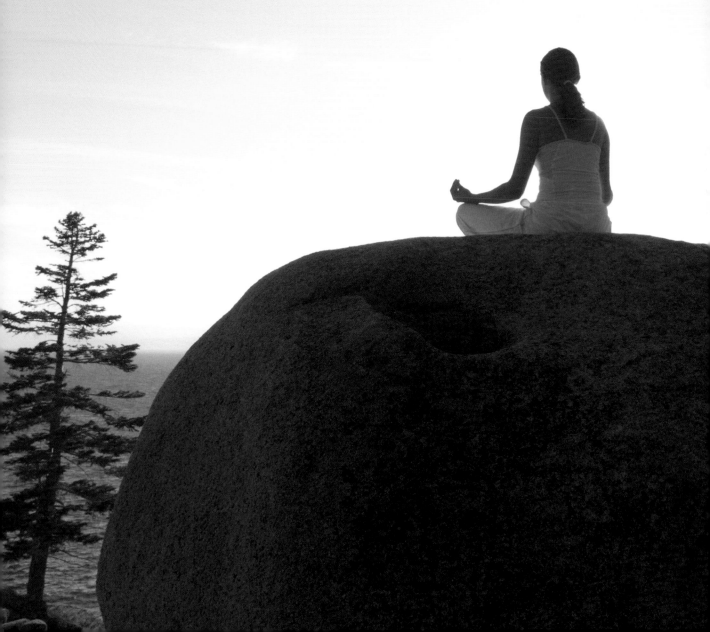

No one knows exactly how spirituality affects health. Some experts attribute the healing effect of spirituality to hope, which is known to benefit your immune system. Others liken spiritual acts to meditation, and still others point to the social connectedness spirituality provides.

It's important to remember that although spirituality is associated with healing, it isn't a cure. Spirituality can help you live life more fully despite your symptoms, but it won't cure your pain.

Chapter 15

Dealing with emotions and behaviors

When chronic pain intrudes on your life, you may find yourself overwhelmed by intense, often negative, emotions, including panic, fear, grief and anger. Like the pain that causes them, these emotions can linger and transform you into a different person — a person you don't like.

Pain can produce changes in your behavior, sense of self-worth and relationships. These changes can also affect your body, sapping your energy and intensifying your pain. The end result can be the development of other conditions, such as depression.

In this chapter, we first discuss depression because it commonly accompanies chronic pain and is a force to be reckoned with. We then offer advice on ways to deal with negative emotions and

behaviors that can lead to chronic pain and depression. The bottom line is, the better you feel about yourself, the better you'll feel physically.

Depression

Pain and depression are closely related. Depression can cause pain — and pain can cause depression. Sometimes pain and depression create a vicious cycle in which pain worsens symptoms of depression, and then the resulting depression worsens feelings of pain.

In many people, depression causes unexplained physical symptoms such as back pain or headaches. Sometimes this kind of pain is the first or the only indication of depression.

Pain and the problems it causes can wear you down over time and may begin to affect your mood. Chronic pain causes a number of problems that can lead to depression, such as trouble sleeping and stress. Disabling pain can lead to low self-esteem due to work, legal or financial issues.

Contrary to what some people think, depression doesn't occur only with pain resulting from an injury that prevents you from working or socializing. It's also common in people who have pain linked to a health condition such as diabetes or migraines.

Depression is a medical disorder that affects your thoughts, moods, feelings, behaviors and even your physical health. Depression can increase your response to pain, or at least increase the severity of your pain. Conversely, chronic pain is stressful and depressing in itself.

Part of the overlap between depression and chronic pain can be explained by biology. Depression and chronic pain share some of the same brain chemicals (neurotransmitters) that act as messengers traveling between nerves. Depression and chronic pain also share some of the same nerve pathways in the emotional (limbic) region of the brain.

Signs and symptoms

Two hallmarks of depression — indications key to establishing a diagnosis — are the loss of interest in normal daily activities and a depressed mood. These key criteria may be expressed in a variety of signs and symptoms associated with depression:

- Feelings of sadness or unhappiness
- Irritability or frustration, even over small matters
- Loss of interest or pleasure in normal activities
- Reduced sex drive
- Insomnia or excessive sleeping
- Changes in appetite — depression often causes decreased appetite and weight loss, but in some people it causes increased cravings for food and weight gain
- Agitation or restlessness — for example, pacing, hand-wringing or an inability to sit still
- Irritability or angry outbursts
- Slowed thinking, speaking or body movements
- Indecisiveness, distractibility and decreased concentration
- Fatigue, tiredness and loss of energy — even small tasks may seem to require a lot of effort
- Feelings of worthlessness or guilt, fixating on past failures or blaming

yourself when things aren't going right

- Trouble thinking, concentrating, making decisions and remembering
- Frequent thoughts of death, dying or suicide
- Crying spells for no apparent reason
- Unexplained physical problems, such as back pain or headaches

For some people, depression symptoms are so severe that it's obvious something isn't right. Other people feel generally miserable. Some people experiencing depression simply feel unhappy without really knowing why.

Depression affects each person in different ways, so signs and symptoms caused by depression vary from person to person. Inherited traits, age, gender and cultural background all play a role in how depression may affect you.

Children and teens

Common symptoms of depression can be a little different in children and teens than they are in adults.

- In younger children, symptoms of depression may include sadness, irritability, hopelessness and worry.
- Symptoms in adolescents and teens may include anxiety, anger and avoidance of social interaction.

- Changes in thinking and sleep are common signs of depression in adolescents and adults but are not as common in younger children.
- In children and teens, depression often occurs along with behavior problems and other mental health conditions, such as anxiety or attention-deficit/hyperactivity disorder (ADHD).
- Schoolwork may suffer in children who are depressed.

Older adults

In older adults, depression may go undiagnosed because it's easy to attribute its symptoms — fatigue, loss of appetite, sleep problems or loss of interest in sex — to other illnesses older adults experience, including pain.

In some older adults, depression may have less obvious symptoms. These individuals may feel dissatisfied with life in general, bored, helpless or worthless. They may always want to stay at home, rather than going out to socialize or doing new things.

Treatment

If you think you may be experiencing depression, it's important that you talk to your doctor. Many people with chronic pain don't mention possible depression to their doctors because they figure that as soon as they get treatment for their pain, their depression will go away. However, to effectively treat your pain, your doctor needs to know that you may also be experiencing depression.

To treat your pain, it's equally important to treat your depression. A better mood often means reduced pain and vice versa. To get signs and symptoms of pain and depression under control, you may need separate treatment for each condition. However, some treatments may help with both.

Medication

Because of shared chemical messengers in the brain, certain antidepressant medications can relieve both pain and depression. Or just the opposite, some medications used to treat pain may worsen depression. That's why it's important your doctor know if you are experiencing depression.

Remember that everyone's different, so finding the right medication or medications for you will likely take some trial and error. This requires patience, as some medications need eight weeks or longer to take full effect and for side effects to ease as your body adjusts.

If you have bothersome side effects, don't stop taking an antidepressant without talking to your doctor first. Some antidepressants can cause withdrawal symptoms unless you slowly taper off your dose, and quitting suddenly may cause a sudden worsening of depression.

It's also important not to give up until you find an antidepressant or medication that's suitable for you — you're likely to find one that works and that doesn't have intolerable side effects.

Psychotherapy

Psychological counseling, commonly referred to has psychotherapy, also can be effective in treating both depression and pain. There are several types of psychotherapy. Each is aimed at helping you deal with one or more issues that may be contributing to your depression and pain.

In these talk sessions, you learn about the causes of depression and pain so that you can better understand them. You also learn how to identify and make changes to unhealthy behaviors or thoughts. Unhealthy, or negative, thoughts are often distortions of reality. Psychotherapy can teach a person how to change such thought patterns and improve the experience of pain.

In addition, you explore relationships and experiences, you find better ways to cope and solve problems, and you learn how to set realistic goals for your life.

Lifestyle changes

Many of the other strategies discussed in this book for treating chronic pain can also improve depression. Stress-reduction techniques, meditation, journaling, staying socially active, eating well and getting regular physical activity can treat depression as well as pain.

Recognizing your losses

For many people, the first step in dealing with negative feelings is to admit that they exist. That can be very difficult to do, especially in a culture that often praises the optimist and criticizes the complainer.

If you're grappling with chronic pain, one of the earliest emotions you may experience is a sense of loss. You may miss:

- The healthy person you once were
- Untroubled family relationships

- Your independence
- Gatherings with friends
- Feelings of energy and confidence
- Job satisfaction
- A sense of happiness
- Sexual intimacy

These are difficult losses. You may feel as if nearly everything precious to you has been taken away. Your natural response is to grieve.

Grieving

Grieving can trigger a number of different feelings. Many people respond to chronic pain with the same feelings that often accompany the loss of a loved one.

Denial

You may deny you're in pain. Or you may continually seek a cure even though you've been told that your pain is incurable.

Anger or frustration

You've tried a number of methods to control your pain, and nothing seems to be working. You've lost your patience. You find yourself more irritable more often. You get upset because others don't seem to understand what you're going through.

Learning positive self-talk

There are many ways to cope with the upsetting changes and emotions chronic pain can produce. One coping technique is positive self-talk.

Self-talk is the stream of thoughts that run through your head every day. Some people refer to this as automatic thinking. Your automatic thoughts may be positive or negative. Some are based on logic and reason. Others may be misconceptions that you formulate from lack of adequate information.

The goal of positive self-talk is to weed out the misconceptions and challenge them with rational and positive thoughts. The process is simple, but it takes time and practice. Throughout the day, stop and evaluate what you're thinking and find a way to put a positive spin on your negative thoughts. Don't say to yourself anything that you wouldn't say to someone else. If a negative thought enters your mind, evaluate it rationally and respond with affirmations of what's good about yourself. Here are some examples:

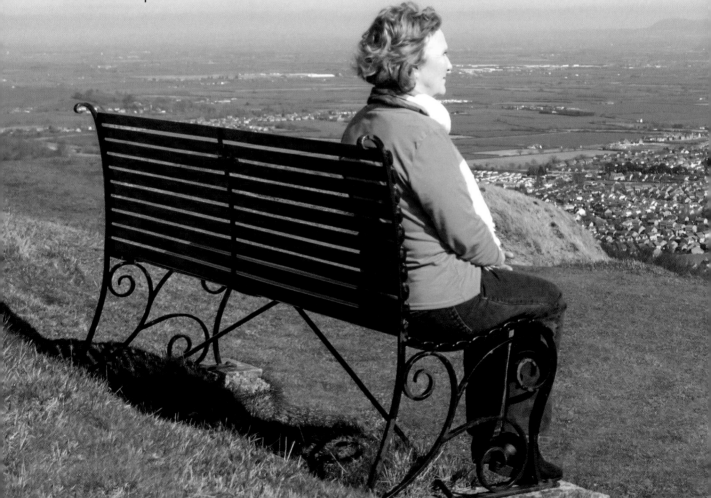

Negative or irrational beliefs	Positive or rational beliefs
Because of my pain, I'm no longer the person I was. I'm no longer loved and appreciated.	I'm worthy of love, and I'm worthy of being appreciated for all that I am.
If I go out with friends and my pain acts up, I won't be able to manage. I'll embarrass myself and ruin things for everyone.	I can enjoy friends and have a good time. I may take breaks from my usual activities, but it can still be fun.
I have no control over my happiness. Pain controls me.	I can control my happiness. I can enjoy life regardless of pain.
I used to be able to do so many things. Now I can't do anything.	I can do a lot more than I thought. Almost everything I used to do I can still do to some degree.
People at work are upset with me. They think I'm not doing my share of the work.	I will do the best job I can. My co-workers will have to learn to accept my limitations.
Medical science can only do so much. Certainly there must be a cure for my pain.	Medical science can't fix everything. Many problems aren't cured but controlled.

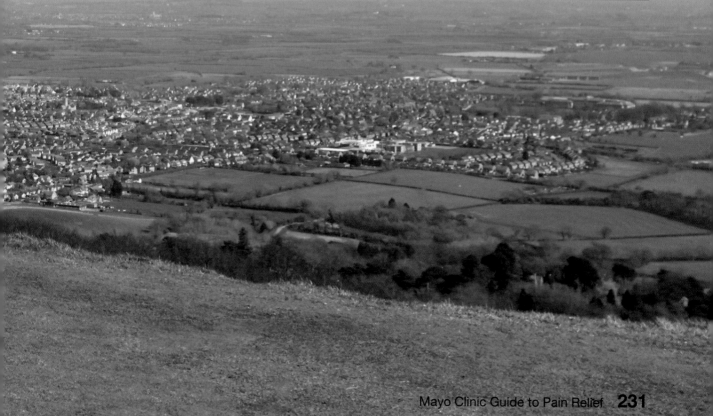

Depression

Over time, you become overwhelmed by feelings of sadness, worthlessness and helplessness. You don't feel like doing anything — even things you once enjoyed — and you have difficulty concentrating. You withdraw from others.

Guilt and shame

You sense you're not the person you used to be. You feel you're letting down those who are closest to you.

Acceptance

You stop focusing on things you can't change and begin to look to the future. You accept that your pain is a part of your life.

As you work your way through these emotions, consider these suggestions:

- Recognize your losses as serious. Don't trivialize them.
- Admit your feelings to yourself and others — especially supportive family, friends and your doctor. Acknowledging and talking about your feelings is the first step toward emotional health.
- Give yourself time for emotional healing, and ask your doctor, a counselor or a therapist for advice and help.

Coping with anxiety

It's normal to feel anxious or worried at times. Everyone does. But if you feel anxious all of the time or your anxiety is interfering with your daily life, you need to talk to a doctor.

Like depression, chronic pain and anxiety tend to go hand in hand. When you have chronic pain, you may fear the worst. You may worry about re-injury, your job status and changes in your finances, or increased pain. Such fears contribute to self-limiting behavior and a self-defeating attitude.

A common fear is that your pain will only get worse. This can become a self-fulfilling prophecy. A cycle can develop in which higher anxiety leads to increased pain sensitivity, which leads to more fear and anxiety, which, in turn, results in more pain.

Fortunately, there are ways to treat and break this destructive pattern. The two main treatments for anxiety are medication and psychotherapy. Medications include anti-anxiety drugs, such as sedatives and antidepressants. Psychotherapy involves receiving help from a mental health professional through a combination of talking and listening.

A tool that you can use to objectively examine the cause of your fears and anxieties is positive self-talk (see "Learning positive self-talk," page 230). In addition, talk with your doctor or another health professional about your fears and concerns, especially if your anxiety level interferes with your daily functioning.

Managing anger

Unrelenting pain, interrupted sleep, unsuccessful treatments, job difficulties and insurance battles — there are a lot of things that can make you angry when you're experiencing pain. But it's unhealthy to stay angry, bottle up your anger or express it with explosive outbursts.

And anger isn't always easy to identify. Mild anger can express itself in the form of increased irritability, or by being short-tempered or difficult to be around.

Whether it's short term and intense or lingering and subdued, mismanaged anger can hurt you in many ways.

Anger can lead to headaches, backaches, high blood pressure, irritable bowel syndrome and other health problems. Anger can also influence your pain. It typically produces muscle tension, making it difficult to relax.

Here are some ideas to help you manage your anger:

- **Identify your anger triggers.** For example, if you know that a particular friend often manages to upset you, prepare for the next visit. Think about topics that spark your anger, and practice what to say to defuse the situation. For example, if your friend brings up a past dispute, respond by saying, "Oh, we've discussed that before. Certainly we've got more interesting things to talk about."
- **Identify symptoms of emerging anger.** What do you do when you start to get angry? Do you clench your teeth? Do your neck and shoulders begin to tense up? Read these symptoms like a caution light — a warning that you're getting angry.
- **Respond to your symptoms.** When you find yourself becoming angry, take a short timeout. Count to 10, take a few deep breaths, look out a window — anything to buy yourself

Types of irrational thinking

Following are some common forms of distorted, negative thinking. A growing amount of research suggests a connection between irrational thinking and increased levels of pain.

Catastrophizing. You automatically anticipate the worst.

Generalizing. You see a troubling event as the beginning of an unending cycle.

Emotionalizing. You let your feelings control your judgment.

Personalizing. When something bad occurs, you automatically think you're to blame.

Filtering. You magnify the negative aspects of a situation and filter out all of the positive ones.

Polarizing. You see things only as black and white, good or bad. There's no middle ground.

some time to let your brain catch up with your emotions and allow you a moment to think before you act.

- **Give yourself time to cool down.** Before you confront the individual who has made you angry, look for a way to release some of your emotional energy. You might go for a walk, visit the gym, clean the house or mow the lawn.
- **Don't bottle up your anger.** Try to deal with disappointment early, before you become extremely angry.

If your anger stems from what someone did or said, talk directly to that person. Deal only with the current situation, and approach it from the perspective of how you feel instead of what the person did.

For example, try a statement like this: "I feel hurt by what you said." That way, you're more likely to find a receptive listener than if you launch a blame-offensive statement, such as, "You insulted me for the 20th time today!"

Responding to irrational thoughts

Life isn't worth living. *Yes, it is. I'll make it through this.*

There's something terribly wrong. *I shouldn't anticipate the worst.*

Because of my pain, I'm stupid and boring. *No, I'm not stupid and boring.*

This isn't fair. Someone should be able to cure my pain. *It may not be fair, but I can deal with it.*

Pain In Control / You In Control

I can't handle the pain. *Maybe a walk will distract me.*

I can't finish anything anymore. *I don't have to finish everything.*

No one wants to be around me. *I can enjoy time with family and friends. I'll talk less about my pain.*

I should be doing more. I've become a burden. *I'm staying active and doing what I can.*

Pain is my whole life. *Pain is not my entire life. There's more to me than my pain.*

- **Find release valves.** Look for creative ways to release the energy produced by your anger. These might include listening to music, painting or writing in your journal.
- **Get a new perspective.** Anger and frustration can increase when you have unrealistic expectations of others or yourself. If changing your environment isn't possible and assertive communication doesn't help, then changing your expectations may help you gain peace of mind.

The bottom line: You can't keep yourself from getting angry, but you can manage your anger so that it doesn't become an ongoing problem.

Overcoming perfectionism

Some people are perfectionists, constantly striving for excellence. These are the homemakers whose house could pass a military white-glove inspection, the master welders who pride themselves on their precision work and the grandparents who never miss their grandchild's soccer games.

This compulsive perfectionism isn't the lifestyle for someone with chronic pain. It's not easy to try and live up to a perfectionist's expectations, and trying to do so can become emotionally and physically damaging.

Before pain invaded your life, perhaps you could work 50 to 60 hours a week with no problem, clean your entire house in two hours and play a set of tennis every Saturday. Now, even part-time work leaves you exhausted, household chores become intimidating, and day-long projects and tennis are unimaginable.

As long as you compare yourself with how you used to be, you'll feel miserable about your performance. Your work won't be good enough, and your leisure time won't be enjoyable enough.

There is, however, a way to keep an upbeat outlook and that's to become a perfectionist at adjusting your goals. People who don't adapt to new challenges are more likely to become discouraged and depressed. But those who are flexible enough to adjust their expectations generally have a positive attitude about life and manage to stay active.

Instead of, "I can't work a full-time job and still keep a perfect house," you might say to yourself, "but I can at least clean up the dirty dishes in the kitchen and make sure the floors aren't littered with newspapers and clothes."

Rather than focus on performance and appearance, as perfectionists often do, work on "perfecting" your character and become an individual who values inner peace, patience and kindness.

Learning to assert yourself

Responding to all of the challenges of daily life can be difficult. And sometimes, one of the toughest tasks is learning to say no, even when doing so is in your best interest. To keep from disappointing others, you do things you know you shouldn't. You spend all day on your feet shopping with a friend. You agree to stay late at work to finish a last-minute project.

This is passive behavior. You put your thoughts, feelings and health aside for the sake of others. Passive behavior can stem from your upbringing and your beliefs about the importance of helping others and treating them with respect. Or it can result from low self-esteem.

Unfortunately, passive behavior and chronic pain can be a dangerous combination. When you continually give in to the wishes of others — at your expense — your frustration can grow, your self-esteem erode and your pain increase.

Aggressive behavior isn't any better. Contrary to passive behavior, aggressive behavior is being insensitive to others or accomplishing your goals at their expense. Examples include barging ahead of people who are waiting patiently, or voicing your opinions in such a way that you intimidate others from speaking up. Often, aggressive behavior begins with "you should" statements, which prompt a negative reply that leads to conflict.

So, how do you stand up for yourself without being blunt or hurtful to others? The answer is assertive behavior.

Assertive behavior is honestly and openly expressing your feelings while showing concern for the feelings of others. Here's an example. "I miss spending time with all of you, and I'd like to go golfing with the group. But instead of playing 18 holes, I'm going to stop after nine and wait for you to finish. I hope you can understand."

Assertive behavior is based on "I" statements. (The word I is used four times in the previous paragraph.) I statements tell people how you feel without placing blame or creating feelings of guilt.

Steps to being more assertive

These suggestions can help you be more assertive when communicating with others:

- **Observe your behavior.** Honestly evaluate your behavior when speaking with others. Are there times when you're assertive, or are you always passive or aggressive? Make a mental note of situations in which you felt you responded well and those in which you feel you could have done better.
- **Think before you respond.** When you want to make a statement or you're asked a question, think briefly about the best way to get your point across assertively,

instead of simply blurting out an automatic response.

- **Plan for a difficult situation.** Think about a situation you're likely to encounter in which you'll need to be assertive. Close your eyes and imagine how you'll respond. What might the person say? What will you say in return?
- **Pay attention to your body language.** As you practice being more assertive, observe how you stand or sit, along with your gestures, facial expressions and eye contact. For example, when talking to someone, do you look at the person? Or do you stare at the ceiling or floor or out a window?

Boosting your self-esteem

Your struggle with chronic pain can result in some damaging blows to your self-image. Some of these are self-imposed, such as your inability to measure up to your own expectations. Others may come from family, friends, colleagues or even strangers.

It's important to maintain a sense of self-worth. The better you feel about yourself, the better you'll take care of yourself. In addition, a positive self-image has been linked to better health and a stronger immune system. Feeling good about yourself may actually improve your health.

Many of the steps discussed in this chapter — managing your anger, practicing positive thinking, challenging your expectations and learning how to assert yourself — will have a positive effect on your self-esteem. As you learn how to control and express your emotions, you'll feel better about yourself and more confident in your abilities. As a result of all of this, your self-image will improve.

There may be days, however, when your self-esteem could use a little energizing. When that happens, consider these suggestions:

- **Structure your day with goals you can meet.** When the day is done, you'll feel a sense of accomplishment.
- **Spend time with others.** Being around people will make you feel more connected and less alone.
- **Talk with a friend.** Having someone who's willing to take time to listen lets you know that you're valued.

Get smart

Here are examples of some emotional and behavioral goals that follow the SMART formula:

Goal: Try not to get so down on myself
When I want to achieve it: One month
How I'm going to do it: Try not blame myself for everything that goes wrong, practice positive self-talk, spend more time with positive people and make it a point to see a funny movie when possible
How I'm going to measure it: Record each day in my journal my mood level on a scale of 1 to 10

Goal: Try not to be such a perfectionist
When I want to achieve it: Three months
How I'm going to do it: Each day make a list of what has to be done and what can wait until another day, learn to relax when things don't go as planned using relaxation techniques, have someone come in once a month to do a full housecleaning
How I'm going to measure it: Plan my day to include time for relaxation and each day record in my journal my anxiety level

- **Find new friends.** Misery loves company, and you may find that some relationships may be negative or even based solely on physical complaints. Make friends with people who have something in common with you as a person, not with people who only share your pain symptoms.
- **Treat yourself to something you enjoy.** Just as you buy gifts for others who are feeling down, you need to do the same for yourself.
- **Spruce up your appearance.** Try a different hairstyle. Buy some new clothes. The better you look, the better you feel about yourself.
- **List reasons people like you.** It reminds you that you have special qualities people enjoy.
- **List things you do well.** Then do one of them.

Behavioral cycle

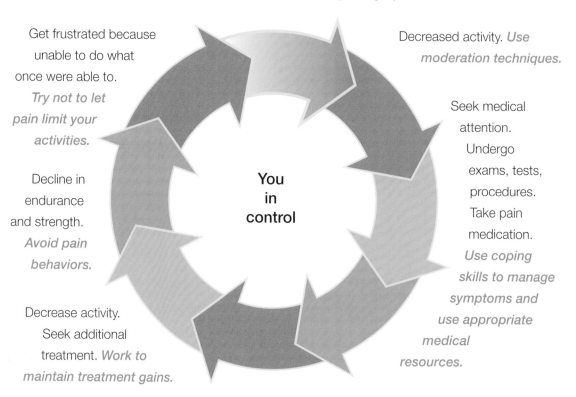

Withdraw and isolate. *Resume family and work roles. Set future goals.*

Experience injury or illness. (Start of pain) *Assess your symptoms.*

Get frustrated because unable to do what once were able to. *Try not to let pain limit your activities.*

Decreased activity. *Use moderation techniques.*

Seek medical attention. Undergo exams, tests, procedures. Take pain medication. *Use coping skills to manage symptoms and use appropriate medical resources.*

Decline in endurance and strength. *Avoid pain behaviors.*

You in control

Decrease activity. Seek additional treatment. *Work to maintain treatment gains.*

Experience an increase in pain. *Use coping strategies — exercise, relaxation, positive self-talk — to manage pain.*

Notice improvement in pain level. *Continue to use moderation techniques.*

Increased activity. Overdo it. *Use time management skills and set realistic goals.*

Emotional cycle

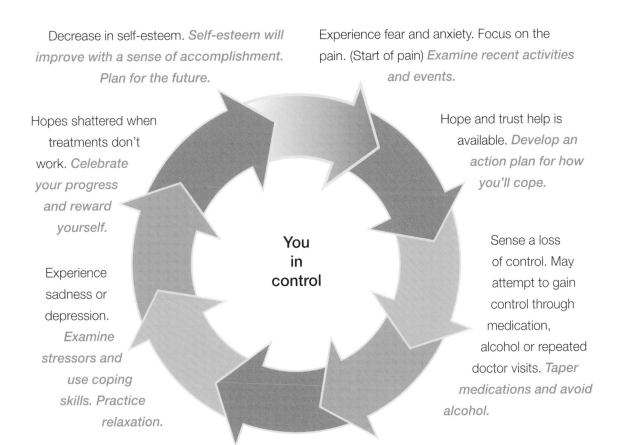

Decrease in self-esteem. *Self-esteem will improve with a sense of accomplishment. Plan for the future.*

Experience fear and anxiety. Focus on the pain. (Start of pain) *Examine recent activities and events.*

Hopes shattered when treatments don't work. *Celebrate your progress and reward yourself.*

Hope and trust help is available. *Develop an action plan for how you'll cope.*

You in control

Sense a loss of control. May attempt to gain control through medication, alcohol or repeated doctor visits. *Taper medications and avoid alcohol.*

Experience sadness or depression. *Examine stressors and use coping skills. Practice relaxation.*

Withdraw. Withhold feelings. *Avoid pain behaviors, especially isolation. Increase social activities.*

Become frustrated, irritable, angry when pain doesn't improve. *Use anger management strategies.*

Feel guilty for behavior. *Work on self-talk and communications skills. Reward yourself for your efforts and progress.*

A healthy sense of self-esteem can improve many aspects of your life. When you value yourself, you're open to learning and feedback from others, which increases your ability to meet and solve challenges. Because you feel secure and worthwhile, your relationships become more positive.

Adopting healthy responses

In Chapter 4, we showed what happens when pain takes control of your behaviors and your emotions. The graphics on pages 240-241 illustrate how you can regain command of your behaviors and emotions by counteracting unhealthy thoughts and actions with healthy responses. The steps that you take to keep your behaviors and emotions in perspective will help you enjoy life and not fall into despair and depression.

Chapter 16

Managing stress

Pain and stress go hand in hand. When you're in pain, you're less able to handle the stress of everyday life. Common hassles turn into major obstacles. Stress may also cause you to do things that intensify your pain, such as tense your muscles, grit your teeth or stiffen your shoulders. In short, pain causes stress, and stress intensifies pain.

The first step in breaking the pain-stress cycle is to realize that stress is your response to an event, not the event itself. It's something you can control. That's why events that are stressful for some people aren't for others. For example, your morning commute may leave you anxious and tense because you use it as worry time. Your co-worker, however, finds her commute relaxing. She enjoys her time alone without distractions. Understanding that you have control over stress can help you develop positive strategies for dealing with it.

The stress response

Remember that your brain comes hard-wired with an alarm system for your protection. When you encounter stress, your body responds in a manner similar to a physical threat. It automatically gears up to face the challenge or musters the strength necessary to get out of trouble's way.

This fight-or-flight response results from the release of hormones that cause your body to shift into overdrive. Your heart beats faster, your blood pressure increases, and your breathing quickens and becomes more shallow.

Your nervous system also springs into action, causing your facial muscles to tighten and your body to perspire more than normal.

In certain situations this type of protection response is good; in others it's not. That's why stress can be both positive and negative:

Positive stress

Positive stress provides a feeling of excitement and opportunity. It often helps athletes perform better in competition than in practice. Some other examples of positive stress include a new job or the birth of a child.

Negative stress

Negative stress occurs when you feel out of control or under constant or intense pressure. In situations such as this, you may have trouble concentrating or you may feel alone. Family, finances, work, isolation and health problems, including pain, are common causes of negative stress.

Too much stress

Too much negative stress on a regular basis can have a negative effect on your health. It isn't good for your body to always be on high alert. In addition to the strain it puts on your cardiovascular system, the hormone cortisol released during stress can cause other unwanted health effects. It may suppress your immune system, making you more susceptible to infections and disease. Stress can also cause headaches and worsen intestinal problems and asthma.

What are your stress triggers?

Stress is often associated with situations or events that you find difficult to handle. How you view things also affects your level of stress. If you have unrealistic or high expectations, chances are you'll experience more than your fair share of stress.

Take some time to think about what causes you stress. Your stress may be linked to external factors, such as:

- Work
- Family
- Relationships
- Unpredictable events
- Daily environment
- Community

Stress can also develop from internal factors, such as:

Taking a breather

Evidence suggests that deep (diaphragmatic) breathing performed regularly on a daily basis can help decrease pain. Practice deep, relaxed breathing at least 10 minutes three times a day and use it whenever you feel stressed. To perform diaphragmatic breathing:

- Lie down on your back or sit comfortably with your feet flat on the floor.
- With your mouth closed and shoulders relaxed, inhale slowly and deeply through your nose to the count of six. Allow the air to fill your diaphragm — the muscle between your abdomen and your chest.
- Pause for a second.
- Slowly exhale the air through your mouth as you count to six.
- Pause for a second.
- Repeat the breathing cycle several times.

You're breathing correctly when your abdomen — not your chest — moves with each breath. When lying down, place a small book on your abdomen. When you breathe in, it should rise. When you breathe out, it should go down.

- Irresponsible behavior
- Poor health habits
- Negative attitudes and feelings
- Unrealistic expectations
- Perfectionism

Jot down what seem to be sources of stress for you. And then ask yourself if there's anything you can do to lessen the stress or avoid these stressors. You will likely find that some of your stressors you can control and some you can't.

Concentrate on stressful events or situations in your life that you can change, such as how you respond to a hectic day at work or how you prepare for a class reunion. Perhaps you can go for a short walk to clear your head or listen to some soothing music.

For events or situations that are beyond your control, such as getting stuck in traffic or an illness in the family, look for ways to adapt — to remain calm under trying circumstances.

How to stress less

It's one thing to be aware of stress in your daily life, but it's another to know how to change it. As you look through your list of stressors, think carefully about why they're so bothersome. For example, if your busy day is a source of stress, ask yourself if it's because you tend to squeeze too many things into your day or because you aren't organized.

The following techniques can help you reduce sources of stress that you can control and better cope with those that you can't.

Modify your lifestyle

Consider these changes to your daily routine as ways to help alleviate stress:

- **Plan your day.** This can help you feel more in control of your life. You might start by getting up 15 minutes earlier to ease the morning rush. Do unpleasant tasks early in the day and be done with them. Keep a written schedule of your daily activities so that you're not faced with conflicts or last-minute rushes (see page 188). Because a pain flare-up can happen at any time, have a backup plan — decide what has to be done now and what can wait until later.
- **Simplify your schedule.** Prioritize, plan and pace yourself. Learn to delegate responsibility to others at home and at work. Say no to added responsibilities or commitments if you're not up to doing them. Try not to feel guilty if you aren't productive every moment.
- **Get organized.** Organize your home and work space so that you know where things are. Keep your house, car and personal belongings in working order to prevent untimely and stressful repairs.
- **Exercise regularly.** Regular physical activity helps loosen your muscles and relieves emotional intensity. Try to exercise for at least 30 minutes most days of the week.
- **Get enough sleep.** This can give you the energy you need to face each day. Going to sleep and awakening at a consistent time also may help you sleep more soundly.
- **Eat well.** A diet that includes a variety of healthy foods provides the right mix of nutrients to keep your body systems working well. When you're healthy, you're better able to control stress and pain.
- **Change the pace.** Occasionally break away from your routine and

explore new territory without a schedule. Take a vacation, even if it's just a weekend getaway.

- **Be positive.** There's no room for "Yes, but … " Avoiding negative self-talk can be difficult. It helps to spend time with people who have a positive outlook and a sense of humor. Laughter actually helps ease pain. It releases endorphins, chemicals in your brain that give you a sense of well-being. If you're feeling stressed, turn on the television or go to the movie theater and enjoy a funny movie.
- **Stay connected.** Recognize when you need the support of family and friends. Talking to others can often relieve pent-up emotions and lead to solutions you hadn't thought of on your own.

- **Take breaks.** Periodically take time to relax, stretch or walk. Relaxation is a great way to combat the effects of stress.

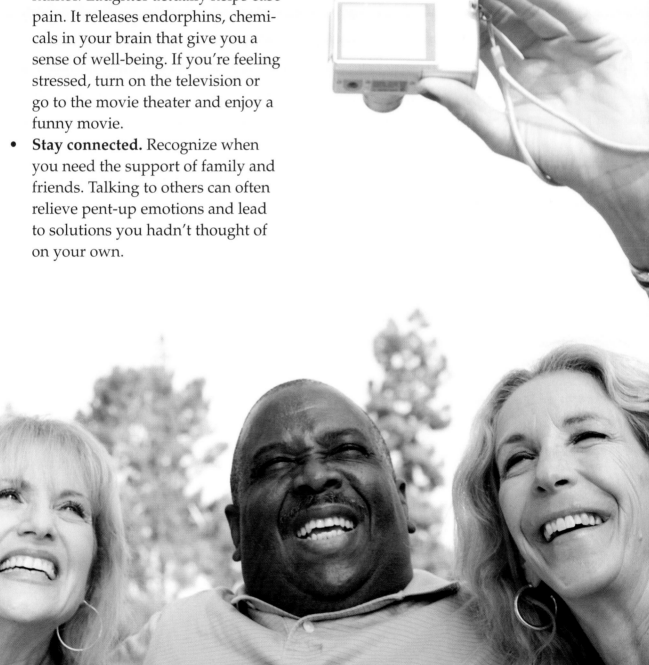

Get smart

Here are some stress-reduction goals that follow the SMART formula:

Goal: Use deep breathing to relax tense muscles
When I want to achieve it: Two weeks
How I'm going to do it: At least twice a day, practice deep, relaxed diaphragmatic breathing
How I'm going to measure it: In my journal, track when I use deep breathing and rate my level of stress before and after

Goal: Make time in my day for self-care, including exercise, healthy meals and relaxation breaks
When I want to achieve it: One month
How I'm going to do it: Use time management skills and schedule the self-care activities on my daily calendar
How I'm going to measure it: Track in my journal the days and times I do self-care activities

How to relax

You can't avert all sources of stress, such as an unexpected visit from family or a problem at work. However, you can modify how you react to these situations by practicing relaxation techniques. Relaxation helps relieve stress that can aggravate chronic pain. It also reduces muscle tension. Relaxation won't cure your pain, but it can:

- Reduce anxiety and conserve energy
- Increase your self-control when dealing with stress
- Help you recognize the difference between tense muscles and relaxed ones
- Help you physically and emotionally handle your daily demands
- Help you remain alert, energetic and productive

Keep in mind, though, that the benefits of relaxation are only as good as your efforts. Learning to relax takes time.

Techniques to try

There are many ways to relax. A number of relaxation techniques, such as yoga, meditation, massage and tai chi are discussed in Chapter 10. Following are some other simple tools you can use when you feel stressed. Work on these relaxation techniques at least once or twice a day until they come naturally. When you're beginning, a quiet place and a relaxation app or CD often help. And remember, a wandering mind is normal when you start out. Just keep bringing your attention back to relaxation.

Deep breathing

Deep breathing from your diaphragm is relaxing. It also exchanges more carbon dioxide for oxygen, to give you more energy. Try to incorporate 20 minutes of deep breathing daily, not just when you're stressed. See "Taking a breather" on page 245.

Progressive muscle relaxation

Progressive muscle relaxation is designed to reduce tension in your muscles. Find a quiet place free from interruption. Get comfortable in a chair or lying on the floor. Beginning with your feet and working through your body to your head and neck, tense each muscle group for at least five seconds and then relax the muscles for up to 30 seconds. Repeat before moving to the next muscle group. For maximum benefit, use the technique once or twice a day.

Guided imagery

Also known as visualization, this method of relaxation involves lying quietly and picturing yourself in a pleasant and peaceful setting. You experience the setting with all of your senses as if you were actually there. For instance, imagine lying on the beach. Picture the beautiful blue sky, smell the salt water, hear the waves and feel the warm breeze on your skin. The messages your brain receives as you experience these senses help you relax.

Chapter 17

Interacting with family and friends

As trying as your pain is for you, it can be every bit as troubling for your family and friends. They want to help you, but they may not know how. So they say or do things they think are helpful but may only add to your frustration.

Because chronic pain is such a personal experience, it's difficult for family and friends to understand exactly what you're going through. In addition, when pain takes over, communication often suffers. You may not feel like discussing your pain or the problems related to it. And family and friends may hesitate to approach certain topics for fear they'll anger or frustrate you.

You need family and friends to help you deal with your pain and move on with your life. Studies show that people with a solid support system — who have family and friends who care about them — generally:

- Cope better with chronic pain
- Are less likely to become depressed
- Are more independent
- Recover faster from illness
- Live longer

Through your own experiences, you may know what researchers are talking about. You've felt how quickly a cup of coffee with a neighbor has lifted your spirits. You've experienced how a helping hand from a relative has helped you get through a bad day. Being around others can help you forget about your frustrations. However, for family and friends to help you, you need to help them. Good communication is important.

Building bridges

Good friends and a supportive family can provide encouraging words, offer gentle but helpful criticisms and lend a hand when you need it. Family and friends also help replace sadness with smiles and laughter. In this way, they contribute to your health and well-being.

Making friendships and maintaining family ties seem to come more naturally for some people than for others.

But even if you're not an outgoing person, you need social support. If your support system is in need of a little strengthening, try these suggestions:

- Answer phone calls and letters.
- Accept invitations to events, even if it feels awkward at first.
- Don't wait to be invited somewhere. Call someone.
- Set aside past differences and approach your relationships with a clean slate.

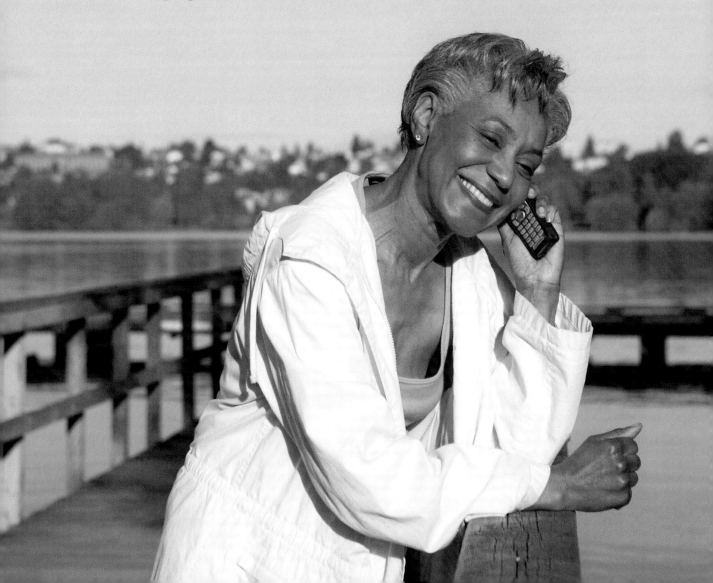

- Take part in community organizations, neighborhood events and family gatherings.
- Strike up a conversation with the person next to you at a local gathering. You could be introducing yourself to a new friend.
- Don't focus on yourself. Talk about things that other people are interested in, and be an alert listener.

Good relationships require patience, compromise and acceptance. Without these things, the relationship can become a source of stress instead of support. Family and friends need to learn to accept you along with your needs, and you need to accept them along with theirs.

It's true that relationships can sometimes be difficult. Your friends and family may want more of your time and energy than you can spare. But instead of pulling away from those you're close to, educate them about your pain. And allow them time to tell you how your pain has affected them.

This will help those closest to you understand why you may not always be able to do all of the things they ask. It will also help you understand how your pain affects others.

Talking openly and honestly

Discussing your thoughts and feelings can be difficult even in the best of times. With chronic pain, the task doesn't get any easier. Instead of continually telling people how you're feeling, it's often easier to withdraw or say as little as possible.

The problem with this approach is that it can frustrate and alienate your family and friends. They may not know how to interpret your withdrawal and they may not be able to figure out that you're having a bad day unless you tell them. You don't have to go on about your symptoms, but simply saying "I'm having a rough day" or "I need some space" will let them know you need time to yourself.

If you're having difficulty talking with family and friends about your pain, don't give up. Consider these suggestions as you take steps to improve communications.

- **Express what you're feeling.** But do it in a positive manner, not one in which you appear to be whining or accusatory. Negative emotions only increase your chances for a

Communicating with your children

Chronic pain is a family affair. When one member of the family has chronic pain, it affects the entire family. Children living with a parent who has chronic pain often have many questions, and they may be insecure about the future. It's also not uncommon for a child to think that a parent's pain is somehow the child's fault. If you have younger children, be open with them about your pain and what you're feeling. This can be difficult, but it's necessary to help your child understand your situation and realize that he or she is not at fault.

Children are often looking for two things: information and reassurance. Talk with them honestly, in an age-appropriate manner about your pain. It's also important for your children to know that you aren't going to die, and the pain isn't contagious. In addition to good communication, develop strategies that allow you to be as active a parent as possible while not pushing yourself too hard. Even though you may not be able to do everything together, you can still be a good parent.

- **Focus on what you can do, rather than what you can't.** Make time for activities you can do together, such as watching movies, baking cookies or playing board games. Your time and attention are more important than the activity.
- **Plan ahead.** When you know that you may have a busy day ahead with your children, make sure to get plenty of rest beforehand.
- **Let your children help.** Children often feel helpless because they want desperately to fix their parents' pain and aren't able to do so. Let them help in ways that they can. Just bringing you a glass of water can make a child feel special and important.
- **Listen to your children's concerns.** Ask your children what it is about your condition that really bothers them. The more you know, the better you can respond to them.
- **Take care of yourself.** In order to take care of your kids, you need to take care of yourself. Explain why you also need time to yourself. They'll understand.
- **Punt when you need to.** When you're having a bad day, have a family member or friend fill in for you at your child's events. Sure, your child would have preferred you were there, but knowing that you cared enough to send someone in your place let's your child know you're doing the best you can.

negative response. For example, if you're frustrated because your friends don't include you in their activities, you might say, "I miss spending time with you on Saturdays, and I sure would like to join you on a hike." Your friends may incorrectly assume you can't take part in recreational events. That's why they don't invite you, not because they don't want to be around you.

- **Don't lie about your pain.** Close family and friends may know not to ask how you're doing every time they see you. But some people won't understand that you may always have some degree of pain. When they inquire how you're doing, don't pretend it doesn't hurt. But don't exaggerate your pain, either. You might respond, "I still have pain, but I'm learning to manage it."

- **Ask for help when you need it.** You were probably taught to cherish your independence, so it may be difficult for you to ask for help. But sometimes you need help. Try asking in a way that explains what's going on. For example: "I've invited friends over for dinner, and it's taking me longer to get the meal prepared than I anticipated. Could you please come over and lend me a hand for a while?"

- **Say thank you — and mean it.** When someone helps you or gives you a heartfelt compliment about progress you're making, say thanks. Don't feel depressed that you needed the help.

- **Talk about what bugs you.** If the flow of communication between you and a family member or friend becomes one-sided, talk about it. Set aside your pride for a while and take the risk of saying exactly how you feel.

- **If you can't say it out loud, spell it out.** Use your journal to express those feelings you have trouble communicating. This not only will buy you time to let these feelings settle but also will give you practice in expressing them when you're ready to discuss them.

How family and friends can help

Chances are your family and friends have asked you what they can do to help you. Perhaps you didn't know what to say, or you felt guilty admitting that you needed any type of special treatment. Or maybe they've decided to help in ways that irritate you. They think they're doing things to make you feel better, but they're not.

When people ask you how they can help, tell them. Here are some suggestions you might pass along:

- **Don't always talk about my pain.** It's easy for friends and family to get caught up in discussing your pain. But that only reminds you of your condition and draws attention to what you're trying to avoid.

- **Try not to hover over me.** Being overly attentive to someone with persistent pain can actually interfere with rehabilitation. One study found that people with chronic pain who were cared for by an overly attentive spouse reported more pain than when they were observed by someone else. Tell your spouse or partner that you appreciate the concern, but that he or she doesn't need to be your servant. You need to learn to do things for yourself.

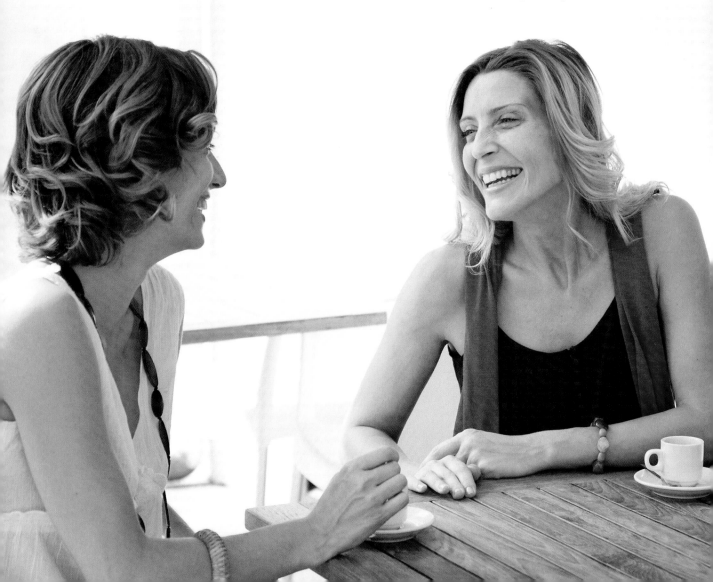

Get smart

Here are some goals for building friendships and improving communication that follow the SMART formula:

Goal: Spend less time by myself
When I want to achieve it: Two months
How I'm going to do it: Call my friend Annie at least once a week, join co-workers for gatherings after work, attend social events at church and in the neighborhood
How I'm going to measure it: Keep track in my journal of the hours I spend with others compared with the hours I'm alone

Goal: Talk more openly with family about how I'm feeling
When I want to achieve it: One month
How I'm going to do it: Set aside Sunday evenings as family time to talk about how we're feeling and the week ahead, and be honest
How I'm going to measure it: Jot down in my journal how family time went — what worked and what didn't — and if it seems to get easier talking about my feelings

- **Join me in activities.** Having friends and family members accompany you for a walk or yoga class or go with you to support meetings or doctor visits can offer many benefits. Being with friends or family members gives you a chance to talk and share time together. It also provides your friends and family members an opportunity to learn more about your need to exercise and stay active.

- **Don't give up things you enjoy for my sake.** Those closest to you may consciously or unconsciously change their lifestyle because of your pain. But that only makes you feel guilty. For example, if you and a friend enjoyed fishing together, don't let your friend sell his tackle just because he thinks you can't fish anymore. Perhaps you can't fish from dawn to dusk as you used to, but you can still fish for a few hours.

- **Be available to listen to me.** Sometimes you simply need someone to listen. A family member or friend who understands that you're not asking them to fix the problem can lend emotional support by just listening to you. This can provide a release valve for your daily stresses. People who feel they have the support of loved ones seem to cope better with their pain and live more active lives.
- **Take care of yourself.** Your pain, and worrying about you, can take a toll on friends and family members. It's important that those you care about take care of their health as well. Just as you need their support, they need yours.

Chapter 18

Staying in control

Throughout this book you've read about different ways to help reduce your pain and improve your quality of life. Perhaps you've already begun to incorporate some of these changes into your daily routine — maybe you're socializing more and walking daily. But perhaps you worry about maintaining the progress that you're making. What happens when you're confronted with a very stressful day? What happens when your pain intensifies and getting tasks done at work or at home becomes difficult?

No doubt, you'll have difficult days on occasion. And there may be times when you catch yourself reverting back to old habits. You can lessen the effects of these occasional setbacks by developing strategies that help keep you focused on your pain management goals.

Getting through bad days

Difficult days will happen! Holidays can be stressful. Then there's bill time or an unpredicted 10-inch snowfall. A visit from relatives also may qualify. Bad days can and do occur.

Whatever the reason for your bad day, you can get through it. One of the best ways to minimize the disruption of a tough day and quickly get back to your usual activities is to plan for it. And the time to plan is when you're having a good day — not a bad one. On a bad day, it may not be easy to think of ways to cope with the problem at hand. In fact, it can be challenging to concentrate on much of anything except the day's souring effect.

Here are some ways to plan ahead for difficult days:

Know your warning signs

Do you get a warning sign when a bad day is beginning? Maybe it's a headache, excessive fatigue or an onset of the blues.

Identify common triggers

Knowing the most common reasons for your difficult days can help you better prepare for them. Think about some recent bad days. Was there a reason for your increased pain? Could it be from too much stress, overdoing it on the weekends, or getting a visit from a particular friend or relative?

Or, perhaps, are your difficult days the result of things you're not doing, such as relaxation exercises, a daily walk or getting enough sleep?

Develop a game plan

When you know a difficult day is coming or you get a warning sign, you often can lessen the negative effects by structuring the day with activities and diversions. Having a written plan can help. Your game plan may include:

- **Maintain a normal schedule.** A difficult day is not a time to overdo it — or to do nothing. Lying around won't help your pain improve or the day go by any faster.

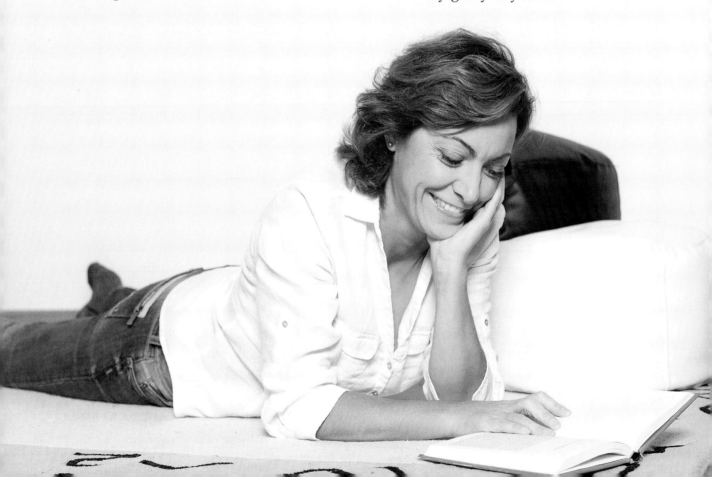

- **Get out of the house.** When you're hurting, it's natural to want to be alone and tend to your wounds. But this only gives you more opportunity to think about your pain. Go shopping or visit a friend who can keep you occupied. But steer your conversations away from your pain.
- **Seek other diversions.** Laughter helps. Read something enjoyable. Watch a funny movie or call a friend who has a good sense of humor.
- **Try to relax.** On a difficult day, spend more time relaxing. Practice your deep-breathing exercises. Use guided imagery or meditation techniques or do some journaling.
- **Keep away from medication.** If you've weaned yourself from medication, don't let a bad day tempt you into using it again. Remind yourself that it's only a temporary solution and that you're better off without it. If you're taking medication, don't change the dose in an attempt to reduce the pain. You only increase your risk of side effects, and the increased dose may not help your pain.
- **Say, 'This will pass.'** It will. It's easy to think the worst on a difficult day, but oftentimes you feel better in the morning.

10 ways to maintain your gains

To stay in control of your pain, use the pain management strategies outlined in this book: daily exercise, moderation skills, relaxation techniques and positive-thinking strategies. The more you use them, the more beneficial they'll become. Here are some other suggestions to help you maintain your progress and avoid relapses.

1. Don't forget your goals
Select your areas of greatest concern, then set specific, measurable and realistic goals to help you deal with those issues. You might be worried, for example, that you'll slip back into your old pain behaviors, such as moaning, complaining or limping. Or maybe you're concerned about keeping up your exercise program. Create a list and check off each goal you reach. To strengthen your motivation, periodically review your checklist.

2. Pull out the contract
Some people find making a personal commitment to improving their lives and managing their pain helps them follow through with their plans. More

What about support groups?

Support groups can provide a depth of help and advice that you might not find anywhere else. That's because they put you face to face with people who share many of the symptoms and feelings that you do. But not all support groups are the same. Some are mostly educational and feature discussions led by informed guest speakers, while others are more social and unstructured with meetings viewed mostly as a time to visit.

What support groups offer

Benefits of a support group vary depending on the group, but they often include:

• **A sense of belonging, of fitting in.** There's a special bond between people whose lives have been disrupted by the same problem. Once you experience how others accept you just as you are, you begin to feel more accepting of yourself.
• **An opportunity to meet people who understand what you're going through.** Family, friends and doctors can sympathize with your problems, but they often can't empathize because they haven't experienced what you have. Support group members generally know what you're feeling and experiencing.
• **A place to exchange advice.** When group members talk, they speak with firsthand experience. They can inform you about helpful coping techniques.
• **A venue to make new friends.** A group member may become a listener when you need to talk or a companion to exercise with.

When support groups aren't the answer

To gain the most benefit from a support group, you have to be willing to share your thoughts and feelings. You must also be willing to learn about and help others. People who are severely depressed and don't want to talk or who have poor social skills are generally less likely to benefit from support groups.

In addition, not all support groups are beneficial. You want to be in a group where the mood is upbeat, the message is positive, and the focus isn't on your pain and symptoms. Group meetings that aren't carefully monitored can become settings in which to vent and share only negative feelings that feed on themselves. That isn't the type of group that you want to be associated with.

than just a goal, a contract becomes a pledge, like other binding agreements you've made throughout your life. If you have a contract, put it where you can see it.

3. Monitor your progress
Keeping track of your accomplishments helps motivate you to continue to strive for your goals. Use charts or some other method to display your progress.

4. Plan your day
When you specifically schedule time for something that you want to do — such as exercising or going to a movie — you're more likely to do it. Also use to-do lists or notes marked on a calendar as a way to remind you of your priorities.

5. Keep it positive
Look around your house and get rid of things that might lure you back into unhealthy habits. For example, is your bed still sitting in the living room to avoid having to walk upstairs to your bedroom? Are the drapes pulled to keep your rooms dark? Make your house feel like a home, not a hospital. When you walk around your house, you want to see evidence of a person who lives a happy and active life.

6. Say, 'yes'
Accept help from others. It doesn't mean that you're failing. The fact is, you need support from others to keep you on track and to help you during difficult days. People who have supportive people around to help them often fare better than do those who

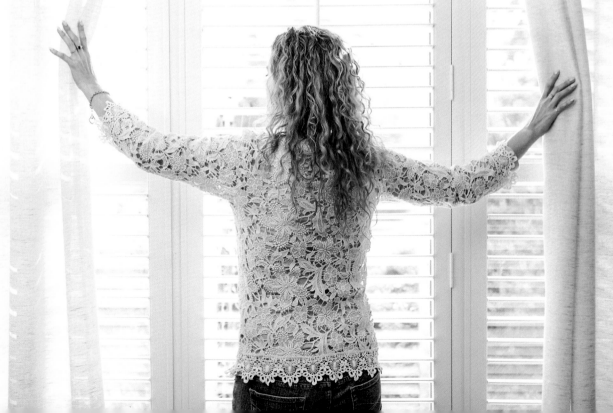

don't have support. In addition to asking for support from family and friends, you might consider joining a chronic pain support group.

7. Team up with a professional

If you're having difficulty following your pain plan, make an appointment to see your doctor. Your doctor, or another health care professional, can be one of your biggest advocates. You might also consider seeking help from a counselor or life coach. Keep this person updated on your progress and obstacles you may encounter. He or she can often help you overcome those obstacles.

8. Talk yourself up

List as many positive statements about yourself as you can and say them to yourself when you're feeling discouraged or in danger of slipping back into some of your old patterns of unhealthy behavior. If you do have a relapse, accept that it happens and move on again, positively.

9. Prepare for challenges

Make a list of situations that could disrupt the positive changes you've made. Prepare a response plan that you can use when needed.

Perhaps you've been walking for 30 minutes each day, but you know the weather will soon be changing and you don't like being outside in the cold. How do you still fit in your walk? One option might be to walk indoors. Or perhaps a local school or mall allows indoor walking during certain hours. Another option is to buy a treadmill or get a gym membership.

Another example might be a change at work. You know you'll be taking on new responsibilities, and that worries you. One way you might make the transition easier is by developing a list ahead of time. Write down all of the new things you'll need to learn. Prioritize the list and decide what steps you need to take to learn each task. Knowing ahead of time exactly what you need to do and how you're going to do it can make the transition less stressful.

10. Reward yourself

Rewards are a great way to reinforce positive change. When you reach a goal or successfully execute a pain strategy, treat yourself to something enjoyable.

Additional resources

Contact these organizations for more information about chronic pain or associated conditions. Some groups offer free printed materials or videos. Others have materials you can purchase.

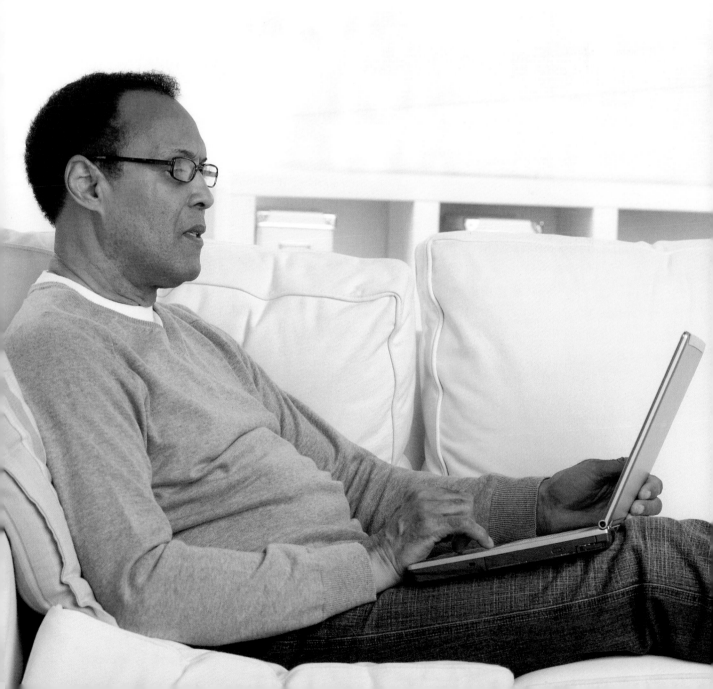

American Academy of
Craniofacial Pain
12100 Sunset Hills Road, Suite 130
Reston, VA 20190
888-322-8651
www.aacfp.org

American Academy of Orofacial Pain
174 S. New York Ave., P.O. Box 478
Oceanville, NJ 08231
609-504-1311
www.aaop.org

American Academy of Pain Medicine
4700 W. Lake Ave.
Glenview, IL 60025
847-375-4731
www.painmed.org

American Chronic Pain Association
P.O. Box 850
Rocklin, CA 95677
800-533-3231
www.theacpa.org

American Headache Society
19 Mantua Road
Mount Royal, NJ 08061
856-423-0043
www.americanheadachesociety.org

American Headache Society
Committee for Headache Education
19 Mantua Road
Mount Royal, NJ 08061
856-423-0258
www.achenet.org

American Pain Society
4700 W. Lake Ave.
Glenview, IL 60025
847-375-4715
www.ampainsoc.org

Arthritis Foundation
1330 W. Peachtree, St., Suite 100
Atlanta, GA 30309
800-283-7800
www.arthritis.org

Endometriosis Association
8585 N. 76th Place
Milwaukee, WI 53223
414-355-2200
www.endometriosisassn.org

Fibromyalgia Network
P.O. Box 31750
Tucson, AZ 85751
520-290-5508
www.fmnetnews.com

International Association for the Study of Pain
1510 H St. NW, Suite 600
Washington, DC 20005
202-524-5300
www.iasp-pain.org

International Foundation for Functional Gastrointestinal Disorders
700 W. Virginia St., Suite 201
Milwaukee, WI 53204
888-964-2001
www.iffgd.org

Interstitial Cystitis Association
1760 Old Meadow Road, Suite 500
McLean, VA 22102
703-442-2070
www.ichelp.org

Mayo Clinic Health Information
www.MayoClinic.org

National Center for Complementary and Alternative Medicine
9000 Rockville Pike
Bethesda, MD 20892
888-644-6226
nccam.nih.gov

National Headache Foundation
820 N. Orleans, Suite 411
Chicago, IL 60610
888-643-5552
www.headaches.org

National Pain Foundation
201 N. Charles St., Suite 710
Baltimore, MD 21201-4111
www.nationalpainfoundation.org

Neuropathy Association
60 E. 42nd St., Suite 942
New York, NY 10165
212-692-0662
www.neuropathy.org

Reflex Sympathetic Dystrophy Syndrome Association
P.O. Box 502
Milford, CT 06460
877-662-7737
www.rsds.org

TMJ Association Ltd.
P.O. Box 26770
Milwaukee, WI 53226
262-432-0350
www.tmj.org

TNA The Facial Pain Association
408 W. University Ave., Suite 602
Gainesville, FL 32601
800-923-3608
www.fpa-support.org

Glossary

A

addiction. An illness in which a person seeks and consumes a substance, such as alcohol, tobacco or a drug, despite the fact that it causes harm.

aerobic exercise. Aerobic means "with oxygen." In reference to exercise, the term refers to the intensity and duration of activity and the energy fuel being used.

allodynia (al-o-DIN-e-uh). An altered sensation in which normally nonpainful events are felt as pain.

analgesic (an-ul-JEE-zik). A medication or agent that reduces pain.

anesthetic. A substance used to abolish sensation.

anticonvulsant. A drug used to prevent seizures that may be used to treat pain.

autonomic nervous system. The portion of the nervous system that regulates involuntary body functions, including those of the heart and intestine. Controls blood flow, digestion and temperature regulation.

B

bursa. A fluid-containing sac that reduces friction between a tendon and a bone or between a bone and skin during movement.

C

celiac plexus. A network of nerve fibers in the abdomen that's controlled by the autonomic nervous system. This group of nerves also conducts pain sensation from the abdominal organs, such as the liver, spleen, stomach and pancreas.

corticosteroids. Anti-inflammatory drugs created from or based on the naturally occurring hormone cortisone produced by the adrenal glands.

cortisone. A naturally occurring hormone produced by the adrenal glands. It decreases inflammation.

COX-2 inhibitor. A nonsteroidal anti-inflammatory drug that specifically inhibits an enzyme known as cyclooxygenase-2 (COX-2). The drug is used to treat pain and may be less likely to cause gastrointestinal bleeding than do other NSAIDs.

D

dysthesia. An unpleasant, abnormal sensation, often described as burning or crawling.

E

endorphins. Naturally occurring molecules made up of amino acids. Endorphins stop pain messages by attaching to certain receptors in the brain and spinal cord — the same receptors that respond to morphine.

enkephalins (en-KEF-uh-lins). Naturally occurring molecules in the brain. Enkephalins attach to special receptors in your brain and spinal cord to stop pain messages. They also affect other functions within the brain and nervous system.

epidural anesthesia. A procedure used to provide anesthesia during labor and some surgeries. Medication is given through a catheter placed in the back. Also called an epidural block.

ergonomics. The science of designing the job to fit the worker, rather than physically forcing the worker's body to fit the job.

F

facet (fah-SET) joint. A joint between two adjacent vertebrae. Each vertebra is connected at the intervertebral disk in the front and the two facet joints in the back.

field block injection. A procedure used to relax a muscle or to reduce muscle pain and inflammation. The targeted muscle is injected with a local anesthetic and corticosteroid. Also called trigger point injection.

frontal cortex. The portion of the brain that's involved with reasoning, planning, abstract thoughts and other complex cognitive functions, in addition to motor function.

H

hyperalgesia. Abnormally increased pain sensation.

I

inflammation. The protective response of body tissues to irritation or injury. Inflammation may be acute or chronic. Signs and symptoms are redness, heat, swelling and pain, often accompanied by loss of function.

intraspinal. Within or into the vertebral column, which contains the spinal cord and cerebrospinal fluid.

L

limbic system. The portion of the brain that produces emotions.

local anesthetic. A medication that blocks electrical signals in nerves. It eliminates pain in a specific part of the body and causes intended, temporary paralysis.

M

myofascial pain. Pain and tenderness in the muscles and adjacent fibrous tissues (fascia).

N

narcotics. A group of drugs that help relieve pain by blocking or interfering with transmission of pain messages to the brain. Also referred to as opioids.

nerve block. A local anesthetic that's injected around a nerve, preventing pain messages traveling along that nerve pathway from reaching the brain. Used most often to relieve pain for a short period, such as during a surgery.

neuralgia. Pain that extends along one or more nerve pathways.

neurobiology. A branch of biology that's concerned with the anatomy and physiology of the nervous system.

neurolytic. A substance or procedure that destroys nerves.

neuromodulation. Electrical stimulation of a peripheral nerve, the spinal cord or the brain for relief of pain. It may be done transcutaneously or with an implanted nerve stimulator.

neuropathic pain. Pain originating from a damaged nerve or nervous system.

neurotransmitters. Chemicals in the brain, such as acetylcholine, serotonin and norepinephrine, that facilitate communication between nerve cells (neurons).

nociceptors (no-sih-SEP-turs). Nerve endings attached to peripheral nerves that detect potential or actual tissue damage. They sense unpleasant situations such as extreme heat, cold or pressure.

nonsteroidal anti-inflammatory drugs (NSAIDs). Medications used to reduce inflammation that aren't corticosteroid based.

O

occupational therapist. A skilled professional who helps people return to ordinary tasks around home and at work by way of lifestyle adaptations and occasionally with the aid of assistive devices.

P

pain behaviors. Responses to pain that include talking about pain, rubbing or protecting an affected part of the body, or avoiding routine activities because of pain.

pain scale. A system of rating pain. Often based on a scale of 0 to 10, with 0 being no pain and 10 being the worst pain imaginable.

pain threshold. The point at which pain is noticeable.

pain tolerance level. The peak amount of pain that a person can endure.

palliative care. Care given to individuals with chronic, often life-threatening illnesses. Care generally focuses on relieving pain or stopping nausea, enhancing quality of life and addressing psychosocial needs.

patient controlled analgesia. A system that allows people to control the amount of pain medication they receive. The person pushes a button and a machine delivers a dose of pain medicine into the bloodstream through a vein.

peripheral nerves. Nerves that run from your spinal cord to all other parts of your body. Peripheral nerves transmit messages from the spinal cord and brain to and from other parts of your body, and send sensory signals back to the spinal cord and brain.

phantom pain. Pain or discomfort following amputation that feels as if it comes from the missing limb.

physiatrist. A doctor who specializes in physical medicine and rehabilitation. A physiatrist evaluates and recommends treatments that restore function in people with chronic disease.

physical dependence. The physical condition in which rapid discontinuation of a substance — such as alcohol, tobacco or a drug — causes a withdrawal reaction.

physical therapist. A trained professional who teaches exercises and other physical activities to aid in rehabilitation and to maximize physical ability with less pain.

R

rebound pain. When regular use of a pain medication makes a person's pain worse instead of better.

receptors. Located on the outer side of a receiving nerve cell, receptors bind the neurotransmitter to the receiving nerve cell and change the activity of this cell.

reflex sympathetic dystrophy (RSD). A chronic, painful condition that usually affects an arm or leg. Signs and symptoms include intense burning or aching pain along with swelling, sweating and hypersensitivity of the area.

regional anesthesia. Medications used to block pain in a certain region of the body without altering consciousness.

S

sciatica. Achiness that may include tingling, numbness or muscle weakness along the sciatic nerve. This major nerve runs through the buttock muscles into the back of the thigh and divides into two nerves behind the knee that run down into the foot.

selective serotonin reuptake inhibitors (SSRIs). Medications used to relieve depression. Thought to work by increasing the availability of a brain chemical (serotonin) that helps to regulate mood.

serotonin (ser-o-TOE-nin). A brain chemical (neurotransmitter) that helps to regulate your mood. A lack of it may lead to depression.

somatosensory cortex. A part of the brain responsible for processing stimulation coming from the skin, body wall, muscles, bones, tendons and joints. It helps determine pain intensity.

spinal nerve block. A procedure that's used to relieve pain affecting a broad area, such as the abdomen or the legs. A local anesthetic is injected in or near the spinal column, preventing pain messages traveling along that nerve pathway from reaching the brain.

stellate ganglion block. A procedure designed to relieve pain caused by overactivity of the sympathetic nervous system in the upper extremities, the head or the neck. A local anesthetic is injected into the front of the neck to block sympathetic nerves without blocking sensory pathways.

sympathetic block. An injection of an anesthetic to relieve pain resulting from abnormal activity of the sympathetic nervous system. The sympathetic nerves control circulation and perspiration and are part of your autonomic nervous system.

syndrome. A collection of symptoms that characterize a specific disease or condition.

T

thalamus. A portion of the brain that relays impulses from the sensory nerves. Sensory nerves enable people to feel objects that they touch, and they allow people to feel pain.

tolerance. The point at which a person adapts to a specific substance, so larger amounts of the medication or a new medication is needed to achieve the same results.

topical agents. Medications applied to the skin rather than ingested or injected. They can come in the form of a cream or a gel. Also called ointments.

transdermal. Entering via the skin, such as a medicated cream absorbed through the skin.

tricyclic antidepressants. A group of drugs used to relieve symptoms of depression. They may also help relieve pain.

trigger points. Places on the body where muscles and adjacent fibrous tissue (fascia) are sensitive to touch. These areas are generally in the upper and lower back muscles, but they may occur elsewhere.

W

withdrawal. The physical or psychological state experienced when certain substances or medications are discontinued rapidly.

Index

A

abdominal exercises, 177–178

abdominal pain, in children, 68

acceptance, 232

acetaminophen, 89–90

activities

    alternating, 192

    asking family and friends to join in, 257

    children with chronic pain and, 82

    leisure, 191

    pain level and, 164–165

    relaxation-promoting, 202

activity

    decrease in, 49–50

    increase in, 50

    linking pain with, 165

    more pain and less, 51–52

    recording in journal, 164–165

acupressure, 152–153

acupuncture, 152–153

acute pain

    back, 32

    chronic pain versus, 25

    controlling, 14

    defined, 14, 25

    trigger, 25

addiction risk

    opioids, 95

    prescription drugs, 113

aerobic exercises, 176–177

alcohol

    excessive, in sleep loss, 61

    limiting, 214–215

    misuse of, 65

alternating activities, 192

analgesics. *See* simple pain relievers

anesthesiologists, 133

anger

    cool-down time, 234

    in emotional cycle, 54

    harm done by, 233

    managing, 233–235

    new perspectives and, 235

    release valves, 235

    symptoms of, 233–234

    triggered by grieving, 229

    triggers, identifying, 233

ankles, range-of-motion exercise, 172

anti-anxiety medications, abuse of, 111

antidepressants

    in depression treatment, 228

    for sleep problems, 108

    SNRIs, 100–102

    SSRIs, 106

    tricyclic, 99–100, 101

    See also depression

anti-seizure medications, 102, 103

anxiety

    coping with, 232–233

    medications for, 102–107

anxiolytics, 106

arm exercises, 182

aromatherapy, 148–149

arthritis

    defined, 29

    forms of, 29

    osteoarthritis, 30–31

    rheumatoid, 31

    signs and symptoms, 29

    See also chronic pain

assertive behavior

    aggressive behavior versus, 237

    defined, 237

    passive behavior versus, 236–237

    steps for improving, 237–238

autonomic nerves, 18

B

back exercises, 179

back pain

    acute, 32

    additional causes of, 34

    areas of, 32

    herniated disk, 33

    muscle strain and spasm, 32

    sciatica, 32–33

    See also chronic pain

baclofen (Lioresal), 129

bad days

    game plan for, 260–261

    getting through, 259–261

    triggers, 260

    warning signs, 260

    See also maintaining control

migraines
    defined, 37
    experience of, 37
    triggers, 37–38
    warning symptoms, 37
    See also headaches
mind-body therapies
    biofeedback, 153–154
    for children with chronic
        pain, 79
    hypnosis, 154
    meditation, 155–156
    music therapy, 156
    tai chi, 156–157
    yoga, 157–158
    See also complementary
        and alternative medicine
mirtazapine (Remeron), 106
moderation
    alcohol consumption,
        214–215
    practicing, 192–193
motor nerves, 18
mouth, jaw and face pain
    burning mouth syndrome,
        39–40
    causes of, 41–42
    temporomandibular dis-
        orders, 40, 41
    trigeminal neuralgia, 40–41
    See also chronic pain
movement therapies, 150–151
muscle relaxants, 109
muscle spasms
    defined, 32
    medications for, 108–109
    pain and, 32

muscle strains, 32
muscular pain, in children, 68
music therapy, 156

N

narcotics. *See* opioids
neck
    pain, 42
    range-of-motion exercise,
        171
nerve stimulators
    defined, 126
    illustrated, 128
    spinal cord and peripheral,
        127–129
    TENS, 126–127
nerves
    autonomic, 18
    damaged, 26
    intercostal, 119
    large peripheral, 121
    motor, 18
    occipital, 119
    peripheral, 19–20
    sensory, 18
nervous system
    composition of, 18
    opioids and, 96
neurologists, 134
neuropathic pain, 26
nonbenzodiazepines, 108
nonsteroidal anti-inflammatory
        drugs (NSAIDs)
    brands, 90
    ceiling effect, 90
    defined, 90

effect illustration, 91
    for inflammation, 109
nortriptyline (Pamelor), 217
NSAIDs. *See* nonsteroidal anti-
        inflammatory drugs

O

occipital injections, 119
occupational therapists,
        141, 175
opioids
    abuse of, 111
    addiction risk, 95
    defined, 92
    effects illustration, 93
    physical dependence on,
        95
    rebound pain and, 96
    side effects, 94
    tolerance to, 95
    tramadol (Ultram) and, 97
    types of, 94
    uses of, 93
    See also medications
organization
    clutter, reducing, 191
    commonly used items
        handy, 190–191
    in healthy lifestyle, 190–191
    in stress management, 246
osteoarthritis
    defined, 30
    illustrated, 30
    pain, 30–31
overachiever's curse, 53
overuse strain injuries, 43–46

MAYO CLINIC

Housecall

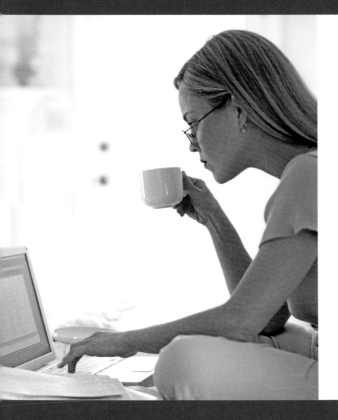

What our readers are saying ...

*"I depend on **Mayo Clinic Housecall** more than any other medical info that shows up on my computer. Thank you so very much."*

"Excellent newsletter. I always find something interesting to read and learn something new."

***"Housecall** is a must read – keep up the good work!"*

*"I love **Housecall**. It is one of the most useful, trusted and beneficial things that come from the Internet."*

*"The **Housecall** is timely, interesting and invaluable in its information. Thanks much to Mayo Clinic for this resource!"*

"I enjoy getting the weekly newsletters. They provide me with friendly reminders, as well as information/ conditions I was not aware of."

Get the latest health information direct from Mayo Clinic ... Sign up today, it's FREE!

Mayo Clinic Housecall is a FREE weekly e-newsletter that offers the latest health information from the experts at Mayo Clinic. Stay up to date on topics that are current, interesting, and most of all important to your health and the health of your family.

What you get

- Weekly top story
- Additional healthy highlights
- Answers from the experts
- Quick access to trusted health tools
- Featured blogs
- Health tip of the week
- Special offers

Don't wait ... Join today!
MayoClinic.com/Housecall/Register

We're committed to helping you enjoy better health and get the most out of life every day. We hope you decide to become part of the Mayo Clinic family, where you can always count on receiving an interesting mix of health information from a trusted source.

More great Mayo Clinic publications

Visit **www.store.MayoClinic.com** for reliable Mayo Clinic publications to help with your top health interests.

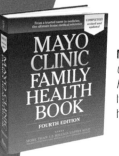

Mayo Clinic Family Health Book
Completely revised and updated Fourth Edition
It's your owner's manual for the human body.

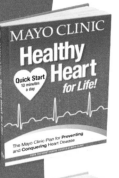

Mayo Clinic Healthy Heart for Life
Start improving your heart health in as little as 10 minutes a day.

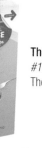

The Mayo Clinic Diet
#1 New York Times Best Seller
The last diet you'll ever need!

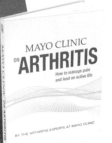

Mayo Clinic on Arthritis
Better medications, improved treatments and self-care tips to lead a more active, comfortable life.

Many more popular titles to choose from ...

» Mayo Clinic on Healthy Aging

» Mayo Clinic on Alzheimer's Disease

» The Mayo Clinic Breast Cancer Book

» Mayo Clinic Essential Diabetes Book

» The Mayo Clinic Diabetes Diet

» The Mayo Clinic Diabetes Diet Journal

» Mayo Clinic on Digestive Health

» Mayo Clinic Fitness for EveryBody

» Fix-It And Enjoy-It Healthy Cookbook

» Mayo Clinic Guide to Your Baby's First Year

» Mayo Clinic Guide to a Healthy Pregnancy

» Mayo Clinic on Better Hearing and Balance

» Mayo Clinic 5 Steps to Controlling High Blood Pressure

» Mayo Clinic Book of Home Remedies

» Mayo Clinic on Managing Incontinence

» The Mayo Clinic Kids' Cookbook

» The New Mayo Clinic Cookbook

» The Mayo Clinic Diet Journal

» Mayo Clinic Guide to Preventing and Treating Osteoporosis

» Mayo Clinic Essential Guide to Prostate Health

» Mayo Clinic Guide to Better Vision

Learn more at
www.store.MayoClinic.com